The Social Animal

Books by Elliot Aronson

1. *Handbook of Social Psychology* (with G. Lindzey). 2nd ed. Reading, Mass.: Addison-Wesley, 1968–1969.
2. *Theories of Cognitive Consistency* (with R. Abelson et al.). Chicago: Rand McNally, 1968.
3. *Voices of Modern Psychology*. Reading, Mass.: Addison-Wesley, 1969.
4. *The Social Animal*. New York: W. H. Freeman, 1972, 1976, 1980, 1984, 1988, 1992, 1995.
5. *Readings About The Social Animal*. New York: W. H. Freeman, 1972, 1976, 1980, 1984, 1988, 1992, 1995.
6. *Social Psychology* (with R. Helmreich). New York: Van Nostrand, 1973.
7. *Research Methods in Social Psychology* (with Carlsmith & Ellsworth). Reading, Mass.: Addison-Wesley, 1976.
8. *The Jigsaw Classroom*. Beverly Hills, Calif.: Sage, 1978.
9. *Burnout: From Tedium to Personal Growth* (with A. Pines & D. Kafry). New York: Free Press, 1981.
10. *Energy Use: The Human Dimension* (with P. C. Stern). New York: W. H. Freeman, 1984.
11. *The Handbook of Social Psychology* (with G. Lindzey), 3rd ed. New York: Random House, 1985.
12. *Career Burnout* (with A. Pines). New York: Free Press, 1988.
13. *Methods of Research in Social Psychology* (with Ellsworth, Carlsmith, & Gonzales). New York: Random House, 1990.
14. *Age of Propaganda* (with A. R. Pratkanis). New York: W. H. Freeman, 1992.
15. *Social Psychology: Volumes 1, 2, & 3* (with A. R. Pratkanis), London: Elgar Ltd., 1992.
16. *Social Psychology: The Heart and the Mind* (with T. Wilson & R. Akert). New York: HarperCollins, 1994.
17. *Social Psychology:* An Introduction (with T. Wilson & R. Akert). New York: Longman, 1999.

Families and Communities Responding to AIDS

Families and Communities Responding to AIDS

Edited by

Peter Aggleton, Graham Hart and Peter Davies

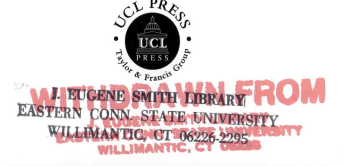

First published 1999
by UCL Press
11 New Fetter Lane
London EC4P 4EE

and

29 West 35th Street
New York, NY 10001
USA

The name of University College London (UCL) is a registered trade mark used by UCL Press with the consent of the owner.

Typeset in Hong Kong by Best-set Typesetter Ltd, Hong Kong
Printed and bound in Great Britain by T.J. International, Padstow, Cornwall

British Library Cataloguing-in-Publication Data
A catalogue record for this book is available from the British Library.

Library of Congress Cataloging in Publication Data
A catalogue record for this book has been requested

ISBN: 1-85728-999-4 HB
      1-85728-965-X PB

Social Aspects of AIDS
Series Editor: Peter Aggleton
(Institute of Education, University of London)

AIDS is not simply a concern for scientists, doctors and medical researchers, it has important social dimensions as well. These include individual, cultural and media responses to the epidemic, stigmatization and discrimination, counselling, care and health promotion. This series of books brings together work from many disciplines including psychology, sociology, cultural and media studies, anthropology, education and history. The titles will be of interest to the general reader, those involved in education and social research, and scientific researchers who want to examine the social aspects of AIDS.

Recent titles include:

Power and Community: Organizational and Cultural Responses to AIDS
Dennis Altman

Moral Threats and Dangerous Desires: AIDS in the News Media
Deborah Lupton

Last Served? Gendering the HIV Pandemic
Cindy Patton

Crossing Borders: Migration, Ethnicity and AIDS
Edited by Mary Haour-Knipe

Bisexualities and AIDS: International Perspectives
Edited by Peter Aggleton

Sexual Interactions and HIV Risk: New Conceptual Perspectives in European Research
Edited by Luc Van Campenhoudt, Mitchell Cohen, Gustavo Guizzardi and Dominique Hausser

AIDS: Activism and Alliances
Edited by Peter Aggleton, Peter Davies and Graham Hart

AIDS as a Gender Issue
Edited by Lorraine Sherr, Catherine Hankins and Lydia Bennett

Drug Injecting and HIV Infection: Global Dimensions and Local Responses
Edited by Gerry Stimson, Don C. Des Jarlais and Andrew Ball

Sexual Behaviour and HIV/AIDS in Europe: Comparisons of National Surveys
Edited by Michel Hubert, Nathalie Bajos and Theo Sandfort

Men Who Sell Sex: International Perspectives on Male Prostitution and AIDS
Edited by Peter Aggleton

The Dutch Response to HIV: Pragmatism and Consensus
Edited by Theo Sandfort

Social Aspects of AIDS
Series Editor: Peter Aggleton
Institute of Education, University of London

Editorial Advisory Board

Contents

Figures   ix

Tables   x

Introduction *by Peter Aggleton and Graham Hart*   1

Chapter 1   Getting on with Life: The Experience of Families
              of Children with HIV Infection   5
              Mary Boulton, Katy Pepper, Sam Walters, Eddy Beck
              and David Miller

Chapter 2   African Refugee Children and HIV/AIDS in London   21
              Martha Chinouya-Mudari and Margaret O'Brien

Chapter 3   Solidarity and Stress: Gender and Local Mobilization in
              Tanzania and Zambia   35
              Janet M. Bujra and Carolyn Baylies

Chapter 4   Gender, Disclosure, Care and Decision Making in
              KwaZulu-Natal, South Africa   53
              Gill Seidel and Rosalind Coleman

Chapter 5   Narratives of Care, Love and Commitment:
              AIDS/HIV and Non-Heterosexual Family Formations   67
              Brian Heaphy, Jeffrey Weeks and Catherine Donovan

Chapter 6   Everyone on the Scene is so Cliquey   83
              Paul Flowers and Graham Hart

Chapter 7   Coming Together: Social Networks of Gay Men
              and HIV Prevention   99
              Kevin Eisenstadt and Philip Gatter

Chapter 8   Observing the Rules: An Ethnographic Study
              of London's Cottages and Cruising Areas   121
              Peter Keogh and Paul Holland

Contents

Chapter 9   Sydney Gay Men's Agreements about Sex   133
Paul Van de Ven, Judy French, June Crawford and Susan Kippax

Chapter 10   Young Gay Men and HIV Risk   147
Danielle Campbell, Paul Van de Ven, Garrett Prestage, June Crawford and Susan Kippax

Chapter 11   A New Method of Peer-Led HIV Prevention with Gay and Bisexual Men   163
Jonathan Shepherd, Glenn Turner and Katherine Weare

Chapter 12   Sexual Risk Taking and HIV Testing: A Qualitative Investigation   185
Susan Beardsell

Chapter 13   Treatment Education: A Multidisciplinary Challenge   199
Will Anderson and Peter Weatherburn

Notes on contributors   213

Index   219

Figures

Figure 4.1 Antenatal HIV seroprevalence, Hlabisa 1992–1997   54
Figure 4.2 Age–sex distribution of reported AIDS cases in
            South Africa 1994   55
Figure 8.1 Relation between interaction and determination of site 128
Figure 8.2 Relation between sexual behaviour and determination
            of site   129
Figure 8.3 Factors influencing sexual behaviour   131
Figure 13.1 HIV: sources of treatment information and their
            importance   205
Figure 13.2 Knowledge of HIV medicine and therapy   207

Tables

Table 1.1	Characteristics of the families	8
Table 4.1	Marginalised rural women: outcomes of a pilot study	61
Table 6.1	Frequency of visits to the gay scene in Glasgow	87
Table 9.1	Men who have been in a regular relationship for more than six months	138
Table 9.2	Participant's HIV status by regular partner's HIV status	138
Table 9.3	Agreements about anal intercourse within the relationship	139
Table 9.4	Agreements about casual sex	139
Table 9.5	Anal intercourse between regular partners	140
Table 9.6	Involvement with casual partners	141
Table 9.7	Length of relationships for men in concordant-negative relationships	142
Table 9.8	Men in concordant-negative relationships	142
Table 9.9	Men in 'negotiated safety' relationships: anal intercourse	143
Table 9.10	Men in 'negotiated safety' relationships: causal partners	143
Table 10.1	City of residence by age	150
Table 10.2	Demographic characteristics by age	150
Table 10.3	Sexual identity, relationships and gay community involvement by age	151
Table 10.4	Beliefs about withdrawal by age and city of residence	152
Table 10.5	Recreational drug use by age	153
Table 10.6	Sexual practice and importance of anal intercourse by age	154
Table 10.7	Seroconcordance and anal intercourse with regular partner by age	155
Table 10.8	Anal intercourse with casual partners by age	156
Table 11.1	Specification of the intervention	169
Table 12.1	Sample for investigating sexual risk taking	186
Table 13.1	Reasons for choosing not to take anti-HIV drugs	203
Table 13.2	Reasons for choosing to take anti-HIV drugs	204
Table 13.3	Attitudes to doctors	208

Introduction

Peter Aggleton and Graham Hart

In both developed and developing countries, the family and the community are central to the provision of care for people living with HIV and AIDS. Shared sentiments and bonds of reciprocity can provide support and understanding when it is most needed, and can help people face the personal crises so often associated with AIDS. But family and community life often has a darker side to it. It is within the family, for example, that people are most likely to experience violence (be it mental or physical), and it is not unknown for communities to react negatively towards people with HIV and AIDS. Discrimination, ostracization and stigmatization are by no means unknown in either setting, and families and communities do not always react with support and understanding to the news that one of their members is seropositive or has AIDS.

This book contains a number of chapters which examine these issues. Each is based on a presentation originally made at the 9th Conference on the Social Aspects of AIDS held at South Bank University in London in May 1997. Since that conference, the authors have revised their papers and brought them up to date so as to shed light on the processes within families and communities that enable some responses to the epidemic to be positive while others remain less so. The emphasis is on the contextual factors which influence the form that responses take, the meanings that underpin them, and the consequences of these responses for social transformation and change.

Terms such as 'family' and 'community' hold a multitude of meanings. For some people, the family refers only to blood relatives and immediate kin; whereas for others, 'families of choice' can be wider, as Brian Heaphy, Jeffrey Weeks and Catherine Donovan make clear. Within families too, perspectives on events differ. The views of children, for example, are often different from those of adults, an issue which is explored here by Mary Boulton, Eddy Beck, Sam Walters, David Miller and Katy Pepper. In their chapter we see how efforts are made to respond to and 'normalize' HIV and AIDS within the broader context of life events. Refugee African children are among those particularly affected by AIDS in countries such as the UK. Many may have one or more parents who are ill. How do younger people respond to this kind of situation, and how do parents 'manage' the information they make available to their children so as to minimize emotional and psychological harm? These are among some of the issues examined by Martha Chinouya-Mudari and Margaret O'Brien in their contribution.

In countries in Africa, HIV and AIDS have taken a terrible toll. Some communities have been so badly affected by the epidemic that few adults in their young and middle years survive. In this kind of situation, how have people responded to the epidemic, and what has been its differential effects on women and men? In two important chapters, Janet Bujra and Carolyn Baylies, and Gill Seidel and Rosalind Coleman examine these questions among other concerns. Both contributions highlight the gender inequalities that structure vulnerability to the epidemic, but both also show how such imbalances are capable to generating forms of resistance which seek to challenge existing gender relations and mitigate their effects.

One of the 'communities' most affected by HIV and AIDS in Europe, Australia and North America is that constituted by gay and other homosexually active men. While often romantically portrayed as an environment characterized by support, tolerance and understanding, the gay scene is in fact a highly complex phenomenon as the chapter by Paul Flowers and Graham Hart shows. Drawing on fieldwork recently conducted in Glasgow, they describe some of the social divisions between gay men, and how reputations (both sexual and otherwise) come to influence the actions gay men take. Similar themes are taken up by Kevin Eisenstadt and Philip Gatter in their analysis of the social networks of gay men in south London. They show how such networks might be exploited within the context of HIV prevention, and how perceived social differences set limits on the attainment of community.

A different understanding of community relations informs Peter Keogh and Paul Holland's work in public sex environments. This describes some of the meanings and understandings that underpin cruising and cottaging, and demonstrates how a sense of commonality and shared purpose can arise in circumstances which to the outsider may appear anonymous and poorly defined. Accessing the meanings, motivations and understandings influencing relationships between men in public sex environments is essential for the development of more effective work to prevent HIV transmission and promote sexual health.

Influences on sexual risk taking are explored in Chapter 9 by Paul Van de Ven, Judy French, June Crawford and Susan Kippax, and in Chapter 12 by Susan Beardsell. Chapter 9 focuses on the nature of gay men's agreements about safer sex in regular and non-regular partnerships and draws on findings from recent research conducted in Australia; Chapter 12 examines the uses to which HIV antibody testing is put by injecting drug users, women and gay men.

In an important chapter, Danielle Campbell, Paul Van De Ven, Garrett Prestage, June Crawford and Susan Kippax ask whether, in Australia at least, younger gay men are at heightened risk for HIV infection, reaching the conclusion there is no clear evidence that this is the case. Why such findings differ

.rom those recently reported elsewhere in the world (most notably in the USA) is worthy of further consideration. The answer may perhaps lie in the structures of community, friendship and affiliation which constitute the 'gay scene' and gay community in different cities across the world.

Peer-led education has often been identified as an effective way of reaching young people with HIV prevention messages. Jonathan Shepherd, Glenn Turner and Katherine Weare describe some of the challenges to making such an approach work in recent research completed with younger gay men. They examine the practicalities of setting up a peer-led education project and raise important questions about the extent to which this kind of work can adequately meet young men's needs.

The last two years have seen growing optimism about the effectiveness of antiretroviral treatments. New combinations of drugs offer the prospect of longer life expectancy and a better quality of life for people living with HIV and AIDS. At the same time, however, treatment regimens are becoming more complex and difficult to adhere to. This raises important questions about how best to help people understand the therapy they are taking and how best to explain drug interactions and possible side effects. In their chapter, Will Anderson and Peter Weatherburn examine these issues, drawing upon findings from work recently conducted in the UK.

Not that long ago, clear distinctions were made between HIV prevention and care, and between individual preventive behaviours and family and community responses. As the epidemic has developed, as treatment advance has taken place, and as the role of the family and community in prevention and care has become better understood, these old divisions are breaking down. We are entering a new era in which prevention and care should be seen as more intimately linked, and in which the power of families and community to support people with HIV and AIDS is more fully appreciated. We hope you enjoy reading the chapters that comprise this volume, and that they offer a clearer understanding of some of these changing relationships. As usual, we would like to thank Helen Thomas for liaising with contributors and preparing the manuscript for publication. We owe special thanks to Caroline Wintersgill at UCL Press for her support throughout the preparation of this book.

Chapter 1

Getting on with Life: The Experience of Families of Children with HIV Infection

Mary Boulton, Katy Pepper, Sam Walters, Eddy Beck and David Miller

While HIV/AIDS in the United Kingdom has largely affected gay men and injecting drug users, children have constituted a small but distinct group of cases since the beginning of the epidemic. By the beginning of 1992, 395 children had been reported as HIV infected (Newell and Peckham, 1993). At that time, the majority (262, 66%) had been infected through blood transfusions or blood products. Since the introduction of screening and treatment of blood and blood products in 1985, no new infections have occurred through this route and vertical transmission, from infected mother to child, has become the main route of infection for children. By the end of July 1995, half (311) of the 621 children identified as HIV positive had been infected in this way (Communicable Disease Report, 1995). By the end of March 1997, the number of children reported to have been infected through vertical transmission had risen to 415 (Communicable Disease Report, 1997). While this number may be relatively small, the results of unlinked anonymous screening in antenatal clinics suggest that, in the London area at least, it is likely to continue to grow (Delamothe, 1995).

The provision of appropriate and effective care for these children requires a sensitive understanding of the effect of HIV infection on their daily lives and of the needs and problems to which this gives rise. As HIV infection affects not only the infected child but also those with whom he or she has close ties, understanding the impact of HIV infection on the family as a whole is also important (Gibb, Duggan and Lewin, 1991). Very little research, however, has been reported on the experience of families of young children who are HIV infected (Bor, Miller and Goldman, 1993; Masters, 1997). Moreover, most of what has been written draws largely on clinical or professional experience rather than on systematic empirical research (Gibb, Duggan and Lewin, 1991; Melvin, 1996). While this has been valuable in identifying the potential problems and sources of stress which families face, it provides little understanding of how families deal with these stresses in their day-to-day lives or how their experience of these problems is shaped by their social circumstances.

This chapter provides an account of the experience of families with an HIV-infected child from the perspective of the families themselves. With regard to children specifically, the impact of HIV infection is to raise the profile of two main concerns. These centre on the children's physical health and on their ability to lead a 'normal life' within their community. These issues are important to all families, but HIV infection transforms them from implicit, background concerns to explicit and problematic issues.

In the rest of this chapter we will outline how these issues emerge in the context of the families' daily lives and describe the ways in which they try to deal with them. A fundamental theme underlying this account is the active and positive efforts that families make to address their problems and the immense resilience and resourcefulness they show in dealing with the stresses they encounter. This theme provides an important balance to much of the literature that identifies the problems and stresses experienced by families, and which implies a very bleak picture. While it is important to recognize the devastating impact of HIV infection on families, it is also important to recognize the positive ways in which they try to deal with it.

The Study

The study was carried out in collaboration with a paediatric clinic in a London teaching hospital which is a regional centre for the care of children with HIV infection. Sixty-four HIV positive or indeterminate children (in 60 families) were seen by the paediatric HIV team between 1 September 1993 and 31 December 1994. The parents of 34 children (in 32 families) were invited to participate in the study. The parents of the other children were not asked to take part, for the following reasons: 13 children had died, 5 children had become HIV seronegative, and 7 children had left the area (5 went abroad) before they could be invited to take part, and 5 were considered inappropriate (they did not speak English or the parent or child was too ill). Of the 32 families who were asked to take part, at least one interview was carried out on the study topics with 22; 2 families refused to take part; and 8 were interviewed but later excluded from the study either because the child converted to HIV seronegative (3 children in 2 families) or because the parents declined to discuss the study topics (6 families).

Wherever possible, the researcher (KP) was introduced to the parents or guardians of the children when they attended the clinic so that they could get to know her before being invited to take part in the study. When families agreed to take part, KP carried out open-ended, loosely structured interviews with one or both the parents or guardians in their own homes. Topics discussed included day-to-day coping; relationships within the family and household; relationships with schools, friends and community; managing symptoms and promoting health; medicines and treatments; and concerns for the future. For practical reasons, where the mother or grandmother was looking after the child, interviews were -generally carried out with her. However, in one two-parent family the interviews were conducted with the father, and in another family, both father and mother took part in the interviews.

The initial design for the study called for six interviews to be conducted with each study family, at monthly intervals. The intention behind this had been, firstly, to allow the researcher time to gain the families' confidence so as to facilitate more open discussion of very sensitive topics and, secondly, to gain a more dynamic picture of how families coped with HIV infection. In practice it proved difficult for both the families and the researcher to keep to this schedule and only 3 families were interviewed monthly over 6 months. Seven more were interviewed 3 to 5 times and the other 12 once or twice. A total of 63 interviews were carried out with the 22 families. Where possible, these were tape-recorded and later transcribed; detailed field notes were kept where tape-recording was not possible. Transcripts and field notes were analyzed according to the methods of inductive analysis used in qualitative research (Glaser and Strauss, 1967; Fitzpatrick and Boulton, 1994, 1996). Where parents' accounts are reported verbatim, their names have been changed to protect confidentiality.

The HIV-infected children in the study were predominantly female (13 girls, 9 boys), and very young: half were of pre-school age (11 under five years old, including 4 children under three years old); 8 children were five or six years old, 2 children were seven or eight years old and only 1 child was over eight (she was twelve years old). All but one had been infected through vertical transmission; one child had been adopted from a Roumanian orphanage and the route of transmission was unknown. Half had symptomatic HIV disease and half had AIDS.

The characteristics of the families are given in Table 1.1. Half the families were headed by a single parent. In two of them the individual providing the parenting was the child's grandmother. In two of the two-parent families, the mother was a stepmother; in a third, the parents had adopted the child. For the sake of simplicity, fathers, mothers, stepmothers, adoptive mothers, adoptive fathers and grandmothers will all be referred to as 'parents'. In two-thirds of the families, the parents had been born in Africa; in four more families, the mother had been born in Africa and the father in the UK. In almost three-quarters of the families, at least one parent in the household was also HIV infected; in at least six others, a parent had already died from an AIDS-related illness.

Responding to Symptoms: Protecting their Children's Health

Perhaps not surprisingly, the first concern to the families identified in the interviews was their child's health. All the children in the study had progressed to symptomatic HIV disease or AIDS and most had been seriously ill at some time in the recent past. All the parents, in turn, were very conscious of their child's current health status and anxious lest they become seriously ill again.

Table 1.1 Characteristics of the families

FAMILY COMPOSITION

Single parent	11	(50%)
Single mother	7	
Single father	2	
Single grandmother	2	
Two parents	11	(50%)
Natural parents	8	
Stepmother and father	2	
Adoptive parents	1	

ETHNIC BACKGROUND OF PARENTS

	Single parents	*Two parents*	*Total (%)*
British/Irish	2	2	4 (18)
Other European	1	0	1 (5)
African	6	7	13 (59)
Mixed	2[a]	2	4 (18)

HIV STATUS OF PARENTS

	Single parents	*Two parents*	*Total (%)*
Positive	8	3	11 (50)
Mixed	–	5	5 (23)
Negative	3	2	5 (23)
Not tested	0	1	1 (5)

[a] Includes one British/Irish father and one African mother.

Although interviews were not conducted when children were acutely ill, about one-third of the children continued to be generally unwell or frequently sick throughout the course of the study. The parents of these children described them as suffering from a range of chronic and unpredictable symptoms. For example, one mother commented:

> She is always sick. Suddenly, her temperature will go up and she will get sick without warning.
>
> (Elizabeth Marks, mother of Hope, 3)

Another mother elaborated on what this meant on a day-to-day basis:

> Sometimes I just wake up in the middle of the night and I just check on him and he is very, very hot. I have to work hard to try and break the temperature down, and he has had so much Calpol. . . . It just happens at night. He is coughing a lot as well. And now the coughing

has got better, it is just this temperature left. I can't really relax at night.

(Deborah Storey, mother of Geoff, 1)

In these families, parents were concerned about a child who was clearly unwell and their child's continuing ill health was a source of anxiety and distress.

But not all children continued to have symptoms or to be so obviously ill. Indeed, in as many as one-third of the families the child was described as apparently well; that is, looking healthy, never sick and very lively. One father commented (with some exaggeration, later qualified):

Evan has never really been ill. He has virtually no illnesses at all. He has had chickenpox but I would say that he has had fewer cold-type illnesses than others and he has never been sick.... Other people's perception of Evan is that he is, exactly as described, a healthy boy, who is bigger, heavier, taller than most of his peers.

(Jon Adams, father of Evan, 7)

A grandmother described her granddaughter in similar terms:

It's amazing she is so well. She always has these little healthy rosy cheeks and she smiles and she is happy. She is so content, she never asks for a thing. She is wonderful, she really is. I can't believe she has got it, I just can't believe it.

(Constance Dale, grandmother of Phyllis, 8)

These parents were also concerned about their child's health but, for them, their child's current *good* health was a source of pleasure or at least relief. Moreover, it was particularly striking that parents whose child, though still ill, appeared to get *better* over the course of the study also found immense pleasure and satisfaction in the improvement. One of the mothers quoted above went on to say:

I never thought I would see him so well as this. I didn't even think he was going to be normal, mentally.... I am very pleased because throughout this winter he has been a bit poorly but he is so much better than before.

(Deborah Storey, mother of Geoff, 1)

Thus it appears that parents' concern about their child's health, though demanding and often distressing, was not entirely negative and could also be a source of significant pleasure and satisfaction.

Whatever their child's health status at the moment, however, all the families were aware that it was precarious and could deteriorate very quickly.

As a result, parents were vigilant about protecting it and very attentive to new symptoms. This was equally the case among families where the child was well and where he or she was not. For example, a woman whose daughter was well said:

> It is funny like that. Even if she has got a little thing, I have got to see to it and rush to the doctor. The hospital doctor says that Susan can be sick and it can be nothing to do with the HIV. But I worry nonetheless, even though he often says it has nothing to do with that. They make me laugh. I tell the doctor she is so well now and I have got my fingers crossed.
>
> (Agnes Oates, mother of Susan, 3)

This was echoed by another woman who described her daughter as frequently unwell:

> I panic more with her than we would with the other one. Because you know that you have got to catch it in the bud, otherwise it all could be too late. So we do worry, like where we would probably go to the doctors with her and they'd have said she'll be all right in the morning, we would have waited till morning, but with her we just keep phoning up and we are not satisfied to wait. Because if she does get anything, she does get ill very quickly, she is really pulled down.
>
> (Jennifer Nichols, mother of Sarah, 4, adopted)

As these quotes suggest, parents recognized that symptoms and minor illnesses are a part of normal childhood. What they saw as problematic in the context of HIV infection was, firstly, distinguishing 'normal' childhood symptoms from the effects of the underlying HIV infection and, secondly, managing 'normal' childhood illnesses so they did not develop into anything more serious. Far from being overwhelmed by this, however, parents responded by taking the initiative themselves, seeking advice on symptoms at an early stage and treating them aggressively from the beginning. In the following example, the mother quoted above describes the lengths to which she routinely went when she suspected the possibility of disease:

> She went to the hospital the day before we went on holiday. She had been to playschool and a little boy came to school smothered in chickenpox and as soon as we see anything like that we have to get an injection into her. We phoned the hospital and they got it in from somewhere and we went up and got it for her. The doctor in London has always said that if ever she comes into contact with any infections like chickenpox, which she could get over and over again, we must get an injection. She has had chickenpox and shingles about twice

now. Every time we see anyone with a spot, we have to go and get
that done.

(Jennifer Nichols, mother of Sarah, 4, adopted)

In the next example a mother who herself has HIV infection contrasts the way
she reacts to symptoms in herself and in her son:

I feel great at the moment. I get a lot of colds and that, and I have
chest infections. The last one was just before Christmas. But I am as
hard as nails. I don't play up. I take my medicine and I cough a lot but
it goes in the end. When Paul gets sick it is different. . . . When he
gets an infection he has to be taken in because he has to have
antibiotics into his hand and has to be looked after and watched.
When he gets them, he gets them really badly. He was in for three
days at Christmas.

(Pauline Jennings, mother of Paul, 2)

Being Proactive: Promoting Children's Health

Thus, overall, parents were concerned about their child's health but dealt with
it positively, by taking an active role in monitoring their symptoms and by
acting quickly to deal with illnesses as they arose. Their response was not
limited to this 'firefighting' approach, however, and for all parents, concern for
their child's physical well-being also meant that they took more proactive steps
to build up their child's health and to prevent it from deteriorating. The kinds
of activities the parents engaged in could be grouped into three main
categories.

First, a number of parents were concerned to feed their children well, as
a way of building up their strength or 'reserve of health' (Blaxter, 1990). By
making sure they ate well, parents seemed to feel that they could give their
child the internal resources to withstand HIV infection and to resist opportunistic infections as they encountered them. The link between food, health and
parental concern was particularly evident where children did not eat well or
did not put on weight. For example, the following mother was clearly dis-
tressed by both her child's failure to gain weight and by the suggestion that this
was because she did not feed him well:

It is a problem, Mark doesn't grow up, he doesn't put on any weight.
Sometimes he has got diarrhoea, and when he has got diarrhoea he
loses weight quickly. Same when he is sick, he doesn't eat and because he is not a fat baby, when he loses half a kilo you see it in his
face and in his eyes. And he is so uptight. Maybe he doesn't want to
eat, he wants you to play but after he says, 'No, no I don't want to

11

eat.' You can play with him for hours and he won't eat. . . . And she [the health visitor] said I didn't feed the baby. I would like that she comes here for a week and feed the baby. I want the baby to put on some weight, otherwise I get angry. She is not right. I cried because she really hurt me a lot.

(Maria Rodrigues, mother of Mark, 3)

By the same token, the following mother was delighted by the improvement in the way her child is eating and by the implications of this for her improving health:

She is very good now she eats. She has two potatoes now instead of none. Everything has changed on her, her hair is growing, she is putting on weight, even the glands are going down.

(Agnes Oates, mother of Susan, 3)

A second way in which parents tried to maintain their child's health revolved around the use of prophylactic drugs prescribed by the hospital. The paediatric clinic generally prescribed antibacterial and antiretroviral drugs, to be taken regularly to reduce the likelihood or severity of further infections. All the parents saw these drugs as powerful and as important to their child's health. Rather than accepting them as prescribed, however, the parents took an active role in evaluating their effects and, where it was felt appropriate, in modifying prescriptions to suit their own child. Some observed that the drugs had 'worked wonders' or described them as 'magic' and administered them conscientiously. But most described altering the initial prescription to suit their own child. The following comments convey the typical way parents observed, altered and evaluated the effects of prophylactic drugs:

She is really only on Septrin at the moment. She was on AZT but she had problems with it and we dropped it. She has been more healthier since. She has put on weight and she did have quite bad diarrhoea with it as well and that has stopped now. So it obviously didn't agree with her.

(Derek Forsythe, father of Louise, 5)

While such adjustments were generally discussed with the doctors in the hospital, this was not always the case, as the following example illustrates:

I was just reading about antibiotics. I am just a bit worried about them. What I don't like about the antibiotics is that she ends up with thrush. It takes ages to clear. It must be difficult to decide what to prescribe to children. I tell my husband that if I feel these alternative medicines are not working, I will always take her to the doctor. But from time to time I think it is better not to have antibiotics.

(Patricia Lennon, mother of Jill, 4)

In both these situations, what seemed to be important was the sense of at least partial control that parents gained by changing or adjusting their children's treatment.

Finally, the third way in which parents tried to support their child's health involved looking outside orthodox medicine and child health practices to alternative therapies and/or prayer. The most popular form of alternative therapy appeared to be herbal medicines, often described as traditional medicine or Chinese herbs. Its use was described at length by four parents, all from Africa, but was mentioned by other parents and may well have been widespread among the families. The following mother describes vitamins and Chinese herbs as central features in her son's treatment:

David is on Septrin. I don't give it to him every time. . . . I give him his vitamins and I use Chinese herbs quite a lot. I give him a supplement which I get ready for him. He is not on AZT; I would never agree to give him it, because it is too strong.

(Alice Elliott, mother of Michael, 6)

Two parents also described homeopathic treatments that they used, and one described reflexology and aromatherapy.

I have a friend there that gives her reflexology. She used to have metamorphic technique but she changed to that and she prefers reflexology. But she hasn't had it recently because she is at school, but we are trying to organize so that he comes here. . . . We have really noticed the difference by the way she has become bouncy and things like her ear infection, she hasn't had.

(Patricia Lennon, mother of Jill, 4)

Perhaps more than any other strategy, the use of alternative therapies conveys the spirit with which families coped with HIV infection and their energetic, positive approach in such distressing circumstances. The mother in the following example expresses the attitude of the majority in the study:

I chose this because when he had PCP they told me, 'We will try to keep him well but the truth is, because he has had PCP, he can become ill again soon', plus 'it may happen in the next few months'. I believed them and I accepted that when I first heard that. But I am not going to sit down and wait. I will do everything

I can. Because to them he is just another patient, and if he dies they say, 'Well we told you.' But the homeopathy gives you hope.
(Deborah Storey, mother of Geoff, 1)

While never completely giving up on orthodox medicine, a number of families turned to alternative therapies to enhance its effects or to provide a backup strategy when it appeared to fail.

Quality of Life: Leading a 'Normal Life'

Alongside the family's concern for the child's physical health was their concern for his or her quality of life more generally. This was usually described in terms of leading a 'normal life' with regard to childhood activities and social relationships and being treated in the same way as other children by other people in the community. As one mother put it:

I would like him to be treated normally. I know there is some thing wrong with him but he can still live a happy life, like a normal child.
(Pauline Jennings, mother of Paul, 2)

Among the major threats to this, of course, were the debilitating effects of chronic HIV infection, acute illness and 'strong' medicines: children who were weak and sickly could not take part in normal activities and were marked out as different. Efforts to keep their children healthy were thus seen as contributing to their quality of life. But the need to take precautions against threats to their child's health could also restrict their lives and conflict with their wishes for normality. This required some difficult decisions and parents described their anxieties about getting the balance right. The mother of a young girl who was frequently ill, for example, said:

The problem is, what do you do? You have got to let her socialize and so you have got to let her catch these things. Basically, you have not got much choice. She has had that chickenpox several times because that always seems to be about nowadays. We can't protect her from everything. We could stop her from going to playschool, but when it comes to school we can't stop her from going there. She has to go. We did say that we would not let her go to playschool, we would keep her away from other children as much as possible until she went to school. But the doctor didn't agree. It is important that she does go among children and has a normal life. So we reluctantly sent her in the end.
(Jennifer Nichols, mother of Sarah, 4, adopted)

The other major threat to 'normality' that parents were concerned about was the way other people would react if they knew the child was HIV infected.

None of the families had themselves been persecuted because of their HIV infection, although several described the experiences of other families who had been forced to move away from their neighbourhood when their child's HIV status had become known. By comparison, their own experiences of rejection were more low-key and limited. Some also described more subtle forms of discrimination, even from friends and family. For example, the following mother, an African woman married to an English man, describes the distress caused to herself and her daughters by the way her mother-in-law acted towards them:

> Jill [HIV positive] would bite into a biscuit and share it with her sisters [HIV negative]. And then they went to stay with her and came back and the fear in the other two's eyes when Jill tried to share a biscuit was awful. It made me so angry, because it was a real fear, they weren't pretending. I said, 'Why are you afraid?' And they said, 'Grandma said that we will get the "bug" if we eat a biscuit she has had too.'
>
> (Patricia Lennon, mother of Jill, 4)

Even those who had not experienced anything like this, anticipated a response of fear, hostility and discrimination against their children if the diagnosis was known. In order to avoid such painful experiences, parents took great pains to keep it secret. This was seen as particularly important in relation to schools, where the parents were concerned that their child be treated 'just like everyone else' and in relation to their own friends whose children were their children's playmates. In the next example, a single mother describes her distress at being pressed to tell a local school about her HIV infection in order to secure a place for her child. While she was very keen that the child should have a place at the school, she was very worried about how the child would be treated if her HIV infection were known. She said:

> How can I go to that school and sit in front of them, the headmistress, and start telling them I am like this, I am like that? What are they going to think of her? They won't like her at the school probably, or maybe the headmistress will keep watch on the child and say she mustn't mix with other children.
>
> (Agnes Oates, mother of Susan, 3)

The next woman expressed similar worries about telling her friends:

> I don't know what to say to people when they ask. I mean, you can't tell them, can you. You can't tell them because they could tell their children, 'Don't go near him, he is dirty.' And things like that.
>
> (Pauline Jennings, mother of Paul, 2)

And the following man described his view on what would happen if his neighbours came to know:

> I think if they actually did come to know then it could be unpleasant. The children around here are not very well behaved and if they thought this was a house of plague it could be unpleasant, I think.
>
> (Jon Adams, father of Evan, 7)

For these reasons, parents were very careful about who they told about their child's HIV infection. Some told the school's head teacher on the grounds that someone needed to know in case the child was ill or had an accident at school. Others did not tell the school's headteacher on the grounds that the child's illness did not require any special considerations. Very few had told anyone outside the immediate family.

But however careful they were about who they *told*, parents were worried that other people could themselves come to *suspect* the child was HIV infected. The kinds of things that parents were concerned would give away their child's HIV status were long or recurrent bouts of illness, frequent hospital visits and regular medication. For example, the following woman described how she had not been able to keep the diagnosis from a friend and neighbour:

> She knew because the girls used to go to the same school as her boy. But Jill was so ill most of the time. You see, if somebody spends a lot of time here, I find it very difficult to find a real reason why Alice is not at school or why she is ill. She was coming to my house quite a lot, so she knew about us.
>
> (Patricia Lennon, mother of Jill, 4)

Another grandmother was anxious that people might guess the child's condition:

> They might guess, I don't know. But I haven't told anyone . . . I don't know whether she tells her friends about her medicines. I think they ask her why. She has told everyone at school that she has got a tube. She tells everyone that. They all know at school.
>
> (Victoria Watkins, grandmother of Ruth, 7)

Most parents were very aware of these potential sources of 'leakage' and took great pains to provide acceptable explanations for any potential signs of the child's infection. Because those involved in playgroups, nurseries or schools had regular contact with the children, where they had not been told of the child's HIV infection, they were the most likely to notice and ask about the child's health. The following mother is typical in the way she dealt with what she took to be increasing suspicion on the part of the school:

> When she started at the other nursery the teacher asked me about the glands, and I said, 'Oh, she has got gland problems', and they believed me.
>
> (Agnes Oates, mother of Susan, 3)

The grandmother in the next example took a similar approach to dealing with questions from other members of the family whom she felt would not respond well to knowing the diagnosis:

> They ask questions, Alice and her brother. But we just say she has her medicine because she has a germ. Which is true, it is no lie. She has got an infection in her blood. So you can't – I mean, I think her family there are so ignorant they would just keep away from her if they knew.
>
> (Victoria Watkins, grandmother of Ruth, 7)

Withdrawal from social activities was one obvious way in which families could avoid such potentially stressful challenges and at least one of the single mothers who was herself ill did raise it as a possibility. But more commonly, families took the opposite view, expressing the wish that their child should not 'miss out' on the opportunities and experiences that other children had and making an effort to give them as full a life as possible. For example, the grandmother quoted above went on to describe the lengths she took to ensure that her granddaughter could go swimming, despite having a tube permanently in her abdomen.

> It is all right until she goes swimming. So what I do now is to put one vest on and then I stick the tube to her vest with special stuff, because she can't have any stickings on her skin. So I put another vest over the top, so she only has a little lump there that shows. But she is quite happy, she goes swimming down at the seaside so it doesn't really worry her.
>
> (Victoria Watkins, grandmother of Ruth, 7)

Where the parents were themselves ill, and particularly where they were also single parents, they were less able to find the energy to make such efforts on a regular basis. In these cases, simply holding the family together and giving the child a normal life, 'just like other children', was a satisfying achievement. The following HIV-infected mother found tremendous pleasure and satisfaction in seeing her son enjoy the common childhood experiences at nursery that others enjoyed:

He loves it at the nursery. He can say their names, he goes everyday until 3.30. If he was playing up and that, I would take him away. But it is good for his development and he sees other children and it teaches him to share. I know he likes it there.

(Pauline Jennings, mother of Paul, 2)

Despite the parents best efforts, however, in the great majority of families one factor severely limited their ability to give their children 'the best possible life' – poverty. In half the families, *none* of the adults were in paid employment and the majority received a range of state benefits and allowances. At least four families lived in overcrowded or inappropriate housing and several more were unhappy with the physical environment in which they lived. Most struggled to make ends meet, particularly when parental illness increased the family's expenses. This shortage of material resources was an enduring problem and source of anxiety for the great majority of families, and in itself fundamentally constrained their ability to lead what the media presents as 'normal family life'.

Discussion

In this chapter we have outlined the primary concerns regarding their HIV-infected children that preoccupy parents and described the ways they have responded to them. However, the impact of HIV infection on families is pervasive and inevitably the range of concerns expressed by the parents in this study was much wider than those relating to children. Parents were also concerned about the conflicts and tensions emerging in family relationships, about what would happen to the family in the future, and about whether, when and how to tell their children about their own HIV infection. Feelings of guilt and blame, of shame and of loss and bereavement were also central to many accounts and reflect another level of concerns and preoccupations within families.

Nevertheless, with regard to their children in particular, the families of HIV-infected children, in common with most families, were primarily concerned with their children's physical health and their ability to lead a normal life within their community. HIV infection poses a fundamental threat to both of these aspects and was perceived as a devastating condition for precisely this reason. Moreover, it was experienced as a persisting, enduring threat from which there was no escape. However well their children were at the moment, parents were conscious that their health was precarious and required efforts to build up and sustain, as well as vigilance to protect from external attacks. Similarly, parents were aware of the likelihood of rejection and abuse if their children were known to be HIV infected and were cautious about disclosing their diagnosis to others and creative in repairing any 'leaks' of information that occurred.

However, while the parents in the study experienced a good deal of anxiety and distress in relation to their concerns about their children, they were not wholly overwhelmed or defeated by them. Instead, they engaged with the challenges they raised and took active steps to address them. The resilience and resourcefulness the families showed in doing so was a theme which ran throughout their accounts. Previous studies which have described the problems and stresses of families have tended to overlook this aspect of their experience (Barratt and Victor, 1994; Melvin and Sherr, 1993). The few studies which have looked at women's experience of HIV infection have pointed to the significance of motherhood in their lives and to their strong commitment to caring for children (e.g. Dooley *et al.*, 1996). This study has taken these observations further in documenting the ways in which they are played out in day-to-day life and in describing the deep rewards and emotional satisfaction they brought to parents. While it is important to recognize the devastating effects that HIV infection has on families and the stresses they face in coping with it, it is also important to keep sight of the efforts that families make to engage with them and their ability to find meaning and rewards in doing so.

This is not to say that all families engaged with the challenges to the same extent, nor that all could carry on coping indefinitely. Where the parents were themselves ill, and particularly where they were also single parents, they had fewer resources to draw on in dealing with the demands of daily life. In these circumstances, parents found the struggle more difficult and were closer to defeat. However, where practical support was provided to the family in the form of home help, child care and possibly respite care, families had so far continued to manage to live independently in the community and to derive considerable emotional rewards and satisfaction from doing so. These findings point to the importance of social services in enabling families to cope positively with HIV infection. Like good medical care, good social services provided needed resources to families and families used them well in creating and maintaining a viable life in extremely difficult circumstances.

Acknowledgements

We would like to thank the Department of Health for funding this study.

References

BARRATT, G. and VICTOR, C. (1994) ' "We just want to be a normal family . . ." Paediatric HIV/AIDS services at an inner London teaching hospital', *AIDS Care*, **6**, pp. 423–30.

BLAXTER, M. (1990) *Health and Lifestyles*. London: Routledge.

BOR, R., MILLER, R. and GOLDMAN, E. (1993) 'HIV/AIDS and the family: a review of research in the first decade', *Journal of Family Therapy*, **15**, pp. 187–204.

COMMUNICABLE DISEASE REPORT (CDR) (1995) *AIDS and HIV-1 infection in the United Kingdom: Monthly Report*, 20 October 1995, pp. 217–20.

COMMUNICABLE DISEASE REPORT (CDR) (1997) *AIDS and HIV Infection in the United Kingdom: Monthly Report*, 25 April 1997, pp. 153–55.

DELAMOTHE, T. (1995) 'HIV infection concentrated in London', *British Medical Journal*, **310**, p. 213.

DOOLEY, M., LAMPING, D., MURCOTT, A. and RENTON, A. (1996) *Health Behaviours and Beliefs of HIV Positive Women: An Analysis of Socio-Cultural Context and Implications for Health Service Provision*. Final report to North Thames Responsive Research Group. London: London School of Hygiene.

FITZPATRICK, R. and BOULTON, M. (1994) 'Qualitative methods for assessing health care', *Quality in Health Care*, **3**, pp. 107–11.

FITZPATRICK, R. and BOULTON, M. (1996) 'Qualitative research in health care 1: the scope and validity of methods', *Journal of Evaluation in Clinical Practice*, **2**, pp. 123–30.

GIBB, D., DUGGAN, C. and LEWIN, R. (1991) 'The family and HIV', *Genitourinary Medicine*, **67**, pp. 363–66.

GLASER, B. and STRAUSS, A. (1967) *The Discovery of Grounded Theory: Strategies for Qualitative Research*. New York: Aldine.

MASTERS, H. (1997) *Parents, Human Immunodeficiency Virus Infection and Drug Use: A Qualitative Study of Families Living in Lothian*. MPhil thesis, University of Edinburgh.

MELVIN, D. (1996) 'Don't forget the children: families living with HIV infection', in Sherr, L., Hankins, C. and Bennett, L. (eds) *AIDS as a Gender Issue*. London: Taylor & Francis.

MELVIN, D. and SHERR, L. (1993) 'The child in the family – responding to AIDS and HIV', *AIDS Care*, **5**, pp. 35–42.

NEWELL, M.-L. and PECKHAM, C. (1993) 'Transmission of HIV infection', in Batty, D. (ed.) *HIV Infection and Children in Need*. London: British Agencies for Adoption and Fostering.

Chapter 2

African Refugee Children and HIV/AIDS in London[1]

Martha Chinouya-Mudari and Margaret O'Brien

I am my daughter's child and I hope to die after her eighteenth birthday so that she be allowed to take care of her younger siblings.
HIV positive asylum-seeking mother

HIV and AIDS together with other chronic illnesses are increasingly challenging dominant conceptualizations of childhood, in particular the notion of children as dependent, passive and non-productive. With the advent of HIV and AIDS, and its impact on families, in particular children, there is a need to understand children's experiences in families living with AIDS and the impact of AIDS on the institution of childhood itself. As recent scholars of childhood have shown, policy makers and researchers have often ignored children's contributions to family life and the domestic economy (O'Brien, 1994; O'Brien and Brannen, 1996) despite the fact that from time immemorial children have been providing care and participating in domestic work. Historically, the presence of 'little mothers' has enabled many marginalized households to get by when mothers or fathers were ill or working long hours (Walvin, 1982). Similarly, contemporary children facing a debilitating illness such as AIDS in their families, utilize such strategies either consciously or by default, as the most appropriate person left, as the above quotation from an asylum-seeking mother implies. However, the role of child carers can conflict with the state of childhood, prompting some policy makers to state unequivocally that children who are carers should be treated as children first, and as carers second.

In this chapter we will examine the tensions for child carers in families affected by AIDS between their roles as carers and their entitlement to a state of childhood. The child carers are African migrant children living in London in the 1990s and as such are a multiply disadvantaged group. For these children the stigmatizing nature of AIDS is overlain by a marginalized asylum-seeking/refugee position, and the general status of being Black and African in London. Daily life is often conducted in an atmosphere of anxiety, worry and sometimes fear, without the support system of an extended family network common in the countries from which they have travelled. Their parents often lack information about local formal support services, linked to unfamiliarity with Social Services and the welfare system in general, and not helped by perceptions of racism from public officers. One of the challenges for these children is to find ways of participating in 'childhood' while they work at supporting and keeping their parents and siblings together.

Notwithstanding global conventions such as the UN Convention on the Rights of the Child,[2] there is little global consensus on what constitutes childhood, or what should be the limits of a caring role for children. Western models of childhood have emphasized play and education as being vital components of the childhood phase and, until recently, childhood has been construed as a relatively passive and dependent state. The importance of children as 'social actors' contributing to and shaping the surrounding social world has become an influential perspective in the 1990s (James and Prout, 1990), with a recognition that there are a 'plurality of pathways to maturity' (Save the Children, 1995: 40). There have been different academic discourses on childhood in sub-Saharan Africa, notably a concern with child health, and a cultural heritage where children's contribution to local and familial economies is expected, and indeed often required, for household survival. Differences in the reliance on older children to provide care are therefore culturally defined as well as related to other developmental factors, in particular the extent of urbanization and mass education in each country. Societies have embedded belief systems about the capacities of children as they develop from infancy to adulthood, about what children can contribute in terms of care duties, and about whether they can be trusted to care for other children. There are also cultural variations about what and at which point it is appropriate for a mother to allow others to care for her child. In order to examine the experience of African refugee children affected by HIV and AIDS and living in London, three case studies will be described.[3]

Demographic Context

HIV/AIDS is a disease of poverty and thrives on social inequality. Broadly speaking, the global distribution of HIV and AIDS follows the geographical mapping of poverty and therefore it is not surprising that sub-Saharan Africa should be one of the regions most affected, given their share of poverty, tropical disease and indeed civil and political strife. Coincidentally, within the UK context, epidemiological patterns among the African communities in London mirror the AIDS epidemic in sub-Saharan Africa. While Africans account for 0.5 per cent of the total British population (Office for National Statistics, 1995) they account for 12 per cent of AIDS reports and therefore constitute the second largest group affected in the UK after gay men (Bhatt, 1995a, b). Like the HIV and AIDS epidemic in sub-Saharan Africa, the epidemic among African communities in the UK is characterized by high numbers of heterosexual and vertical transmissions, in contrast to the predominant homosexual pattern in the UK.

The geographical distribution of children affected by HIV and AIDS in the UK follows the epidemiological distribution of HIV and AIDS adult cases, with a majority of cases occurring in the metropolitan areas, particularly in the London regions. Estimates suggest there are likely to be over 3,000 children affected by AIDS in the UK, including 2,000 under the age of 10, and that these numbers are on the increase (Imrie and Coombes, 1995). The most affected age group are children under age 10 years. A large proportion of HIV-affected children in the Thames region are from Black and ethnic minority communities and many of them have parents who are African-born and/or recent immigrants or asylum seekers in this country (Imrie and Coombes, 1995: 11).

London's Black African Children

Twelve per cent of children in the UK live in London, with 40 per cent of all children from ethnic minority families living in London (Lesser, 1995). The 1991 census data indicates that nearly 80 per cent of Black African children in the UK live in London. The relatively low proportions of Black Africans, Bangladeshis and other ethnic Asians born in the UK (according to 1991 census) indicates that these populations are recently arrived in the UK, although this is increasingly less true for children from established ethnic minority groups. Census data (1991) also indicates that a higher proportion of Black African children live in families involving 'other adults' (who may not be parents) than White children, and that there is a higher proportion of Black African children living in one-parent families than is the case for children in White families. Children's living conditions and circumstances have an impact on health, with census data (1991) indicating that the highest levels of long-standing illnesses are found among London-based Black African children when compared to other groups of children living in London. There is, however, notable diversity and difference between and within the localities where ethnic minority children reside in London; with Southwark, Lambeth and Hackney having the highest proportion of Black African children (Lesser, 1995).

Refugee Communities and HIV-related Risk

According to the 1951 Geneva Convention, refugees are

> persons who are outside their country of origin because of a well founded fear of persecution for reasons of race, religion, nationality, membership of a particular social group or political opinion and unable or owing to such a fear, unwilling to avail himself of the protection of that country; or who, not having a nationality and being

outside of his former habitual residence . . . is unable or, owing to that fear is unable to return to it.

Refugee children are the dependents (under the age of 18) of adults who fall under the definition of refugee or an asylum seeker in the UK (although persons under the age of 18 can claim refugee status in their own right, e.g. as unaccompanied refugee or asylum-seeking children). In 1994 the United Nations High Commission for Refugees estimated that approximately 75 per cent of the world's refugees are women and children (United Nations High Commission for Refugees, 1994). But in the UK context there has been confusion about the terms 'refugee' and 'asylum seeker'. Formally, an asylum seeker is someone whose application is pending Home Office approval for refugee status. The children reported in this chapter often fell between formal legal categories.

According to the Refugee Council, HIV spreads fastest in conditions of poverty, powerlessness, war and social instability, precisely the conditions that create refugees. In situations of war and civil strife, HIV prevention strategies are disrupted or completely collapsed: women and girls run an increased risk of violence, including rape and coercive sex, with associated risks of HIV transmission (Maharaj *et al.*, 1996). The dislocation of communities breaks familial bonds and relationships and thereby increases the risk of transmission as new relationships are formed, or as powerless members of the community are put at risk of contracting HIV through sexual violence. As Dodge-Cole (1990) has noted, war and civil strife severely disrupt essential medical supplies, with hospitals often unable to carry out basic measures such as the sterilization of medical equipment and the screening of blood supplies. Moreover, survival strategies in the flight to safety may put some refugees at risk of contracting HIV. These strategies may include the exchange of sexual favours for fundamental needs such as food and safety.

The African communities most affected by HIV and AIDS in London tend to be those of East African origin, including the Ugandan community and increasing numbers of Zairians and Rwandans. East African families tend also to have had a history of involvement in civil and political strife.

Case Studies

Three case studies generated in the pilot phase of the HIV and Family Project with which we are involved will now be described. The larger study will include a large-scale survey of London-based families in which children affected by HIV and AIDS live, as well as in-depth interviews with a subsample. Children in the three cases range in age from 9 to 18 years. It is notable that a majority of the cases generated from the pilot work are girls, in line with the findings by Newton and Becker (1996), who found that 11 out of the 12 young carers in their sample in Southwark, London, were female.

Beauty

Beauty is a 14-year-old refugee girl who lives with her father who has an AIDS-defining illness. The family lives in a two-bedroomed council house. When Beauty was 10, her father who was in the Rwandan Army had to flee the country and leave Beauty and her mother in Rwanda. While in Rwanda, her mother was shot dead during the political unrest. Soon after her mother's death, Beauty, who was now staying with her mother's sister, had to leave the country to come and join her father in London. On arrival in London, Beauty had to contend with the double shock of having lost her mother and also having to see her father quite ill. Beauty's family have no other kin in the UK, a fact that at times stresses Beauty as she misses her family in Rwanda and some of her friends.

Because of limited kin networks, Beauty is now caring for her father, by helping with cooking, cleaning and laundry, organizing bills, postage, etc. There is a home help from the local authority who comes to assist the family three days a week. Although registered at the local school, Beauty is known to the school for poor punctuality and poor grades, factors that have made her hate school, a situation aggravated by communication difficulties as English is not her first language. Furthermore, she has been taunted at school because of her accent. Beauty has no time to engage with other children of her age because she worries that her father may want some assistance while she is out. Her father does not want to access any more services as he fears that his confidentiality might be breached; he is not yet ready to explain to his daughter the cause of his continuous illness. Furthermore, Beauty's father does not know how he is going to explain to his daughter the different people coming to offer assistance to the family. Beauty's father is stressed by the role that his daughter plays. As he described it:

> It is a pity that my child is no longer a child. . . . For me as a father, the stress comes when my sense of fatherhood is challenged. I am no longer a *father* any more. My daughter, in her role, is challenging me to continue being a father.

Karen

Karen is a 15-year-old Zairian girl who lives with her mother and two younger siblings, Henry (age 4) and Mavis (age 7). Karen's mother, Henry and Mavis are all HIV positive; Karen is HIV negative. This illustrates an age-differentiated disease pattern among siblings of HIV families, where older siblings may be negative and the more recently born may be positive. The family does not know whether Karen's father is still alive, as he 'disappeared' while the family was still in Zaire. Karen's mother has an AIDS-defining illness. Karen is the main carer in the home, although there is some help from a voluntary organization to complement her care. Karen looks after her mother when she is unwell and the tasks vary in relation to her mother's health at the time. Karen's main care duties involve taking her siblings to school, preparing food, cleaning, personal care for the younger siblings and other domestic tasks. Her caring tasks are intensified when her mother is unwell. The most difficult times are when her siblings are unwell and she has to contend with being in a household where a majority of the members are sick. Karen has not been told the cause of illness in the family, although she has been 'guessing' at what her mother and siblings could be suffering from, at times wondering why she has not been hospitalized or unwell like her siblings, feelings that are compounded by fear and guilt. It is difficult for Karen to plan to go out with friends as her mother's health is, as Karen puts it, 'up and down'. Karen cannot go out to play as she feels responsible for the family's well-being, 'I cannot go out just in case my family needs me.' Karen also finds school difficult as at times she gets to school late and at times she fails to concentrate.

Sarah

Sarah is a 9-year-old girl who lives with her mother and young brother, Sam (age 2) in a temporary one-bed flat. Both mother and Sam have an AIDS-defining illness and have been hospitalized on a number of occasions. The family fled Zaire and left their father and two older siblings (boys), who at the time were staying with their grandparents in another area when Sarah and her mother, then pregnant, managed to come to London. The family in London do not know whether the father and the two siblings are still alive. Efforts to write or make contact with the family in Zaire have been in vain. There is growing fear and uncertainty among Sarah and her family in London that their father and her brothers have either moved from where the old residence was, or are dead. Sarah often thinks of and misses her father, brothers and her other biological and social kin. When her mother is unwell, Sarah 'helps' with the housework, and with feeding and bathing Sam. She spends a lot of time caring for her mother, who is bedridden, although the family has a volunteer who helps with daily tasks. The family are entitled to only limited benefits as their immigration status is still under investigation by the Home Office. Sarah knows the cause of her mother's illness and the impending deaths in the family. When not at school, Sarah wants to be with her mother all the time because, as Sarah puts it, 'If I leave her, she will die.'

Themes

Lack of Extended Family Network: Children as Carers

AIDS has been described as a 'family burden', thus signifying the central role of the family in the management of disease (Ankrah, 1993). In Africa the role of the family can be clearly seen in the absorption of AIDS orphans within the extended family structure, providing care and support to family members. Also in their caring roles in Africa, children would be supervised and offered support and guidance by adults within their extended family networks (Chinouya-Mudari, 1997). For African families affected by HIV/AIDS in London, there is a complicated and varied response due to the diversity and differences between and within various African communities and their reactions to the AIDS epidemic. Working within that framework of diversity, African asylum-seeking families affected by HIV/AIDS, being in most cases first-generation immigrants to the UK, tend to have limited family networks and support, thus leading to families being resourceful in the management of illness and disease associated with AIDS. However, lack of extended family support means that the burden of caregiving cannot be shared by the family but instead is increasingly devolved to the childhood generation.

Children who care perform a wide range of duties such as basic house-hold tasks, childcare, personal care for ill relatives, or being a pillar of support to parents and other siblings who are going through emotional and physical turmoil as a result of AIDS or HIV. Caregiving is a complex process involving the emotional or psychological dimension of 'caring about' as well as the provision of practical assistance which is 'caring for'. The fusion of 'caring about' with 'caring for', between love and labour, often intensifies the stress experienced by the family caregiver, especially women (Lewis and Meredith, 1988). In this instance it is in line with gender expectations in family care for African female, young carers in the family. Moreover, actions that are perceived as supportive by the receiver may be stressful to the provider (the caregiver's burden). For African asylum-seeking children providing family care, the caregiver's burden is augmented by the psychological stress and trauma of watching parents and siblings deterio-rate and die. Sarah is aware of her mother's impending death, and demon-strates her extreme stress in the interview; as she points out, 'If I leave her, she will die.' Sarah would rather be with her mother than play with friends, as she genuinely believes that by being with her mother she is able to prevent the impending death. In stressful conditions, many children age 9, and indeed many adults, are not able to fully differentiate formal patterns of causation, so they may implicate themselves as an active agent in parental death, disease or divorce.

Patterns of Disclosure

Anecdotal evidence indicates that a significant proportion of African refugee children affected by HIV and AIDS are unaware of the cause of illness in the family, thus raising the dilemma faced by many parents about whether to disclose the cause of illness to the children in the family: disclosure not only to the children who are carers but also to children like Sam, Henry and Mavis, who are directly infected. Both Beauty and Karen are unaware of the cause of illness in the family; in Beauty's case this is intensifying her caring role, as her father does not wish to access any more services. Like a number of other parents affected by HIV and AIDS, Beauty's father is anxious about confidentiality as he is not sure about how he would explain to his daughter the increased care from different agencies. He is also anxious that the new carers may breach his confidentiality. Parents facing the debate around disclosure are also going through a series of dilemmas; Beauty's father is stressed by the role his daughter is playing but feels helpless to restore her right to childhood.

Newton and Becker (1996) noted that children affected and caring for families affected by HIV and AIDS suffer from 'courtesy stigma', or stigma by association. Children such as Sarah, who are aware of the cause of illness, cannot take pride in their caring role because of the stigma associated with HIV/AIDS. Lack of information about the support services available, unresolved immigration status, the stigma associated with HIV/AIDS, and fear that the disclosure of family circumstances (in this instance the caring roles of the child, HIV in the family, etc.) may lead to the children being 'taken away' (by social services), these are some of the reasons cited by the families for not accessing services. Anecdotal evidence indicates that some parents feel there is also a lack of clear school policies concerning confidentiality issues related to HIV in families, making it difficult for families to explain to the school about the child's circumstances.

Loss of Childhood

Caring poses a threat to children who are carers as it affects their psychosocial development as a result of exclusion, isolation and interference with education. For African children affected and caring for families affected by HIV and AIDS, loss of childhood is compounded by language barriers which can lead to a 'problem in a vacuum', as such children may find it difficult to express the stress they are going through as a result of their caring roles and AIDS in the family. Notwithstanding the cultural diversity between and within African children, the need to communicate stress associated with caring roles may be compounded by the fact that, culturally, the disclosure of family circumstances to 'strangers' may be inappropriate, more so given the children's personal trajectories and life experiences as refugees.

These three case studies clearly show the loss of important dimensions of childhood, especially time to play and time to interact with other children. Parents' concerns about confidentiality, and the stigma associated with HIV/AIDS, can result in their limiting the number of associations that their children have. These cases also show how young carers set personal limits on their social worlds, trying to keep the 'family secret' even if they are not fully aware of the reasons why. The stresses and strains of childhood caring can prove too much for some young carers: two of the twelve young carers in a recent study in Southwark, London, mentioned taking an overdose in the past two years, and some of the carers identified the stress of their caring role as a contributing factor (Newton and Becker, 1996).

Missing School

In line with the findings by Newton and Becker (1996) – one in four young carers of compulsory school age miss school as a result of their caring work. Lateness has been an issue for Karen as she has to put the needs of her family above getting to school on time. Caring also affects her doing homework or participating in after-school activities, leading ultimately in her case to lateness, poor attendance and low grades. Moreover, for most African refugee children living in London, English is not their first language. Children affected by HIV and AIDS are more likely to suffer educational disadvantages (Imrie and Coombes, 1995). English was not the first language for Karen, Beauty and Sarah, and all described how language difficulties placed constraints on both their educational and social worlds.

Multiple Family Disruptions and Multiple Losses

The transitions and flows into different family types are a continuous source of stress and insecurity for children affected by AIDS. Many have memories of living with the whole family and being close to a wider kin group in Africa before the disruptions and traumas associated with war. Due to the effects of war, a majority of such children are separated from one of their parents, usually the father, and sometimes their siblings; they suffer from the stress that accompanies loss and living with uncertainty about the well-being of the extended family in Africa, as demonstrated by Sarah. Remembering this time, Sarah's mother said:

> Because of the war situation, I only managed to bring with me my youngest child, who was with me at the time we managed to escape. I was pregnant at the time. My other two were being looked after and helping their grandmother in another area. We are all worried as to

whether they are still alive or not, as efforts to contact them have been unfruitful. . . . As for my husband, I do not know if he is still alive or not.

Parental and sibling separation brings with it feelings of loss, grief, anger and guilt in the family, and these are compounded by the pressures of adapting to a new lifestyle and status in the UK. Comparatively, within the UK context, where rising divorce rates, separations and births outside marriage are a major cause of lone parenthood, a majority of African refugee children affected by HIV and AIDS are experiencing lone parenthood due to death of a parent either due to political and civil turmoil, deaths or stresses related to HIV in the family, and the general impact of migration and its legal implications. Family life therefore becomes a transient and fluid social phenomenon. Because there is no cure for AIDS at the moment, many children affected by AIDS face future disruptions through the death of siblings, parents or other family members, and sometimes orphanhood.

Policy and Practice Implications

Young African carers, and indeed other children who are caring for their families, are children with rights and needs that are legally protected, globally through the United Nations Convention on the Rights of the Child and locally in the UK through the Children Act (Department of Health, 1989). According to Section 17 of the Children Act, African refugee children are deemed 'children in need'. A child is in need if:

(a) he is unlikely to achieve or maintain, or to have the opportunity of achieving or maintaining, a reasonable standard of health or development without the provision of services by a local authority under this part; (b) his health development is likely to be significantly impaired or further impaired; (c) or if the child has a disability.

The level of need for each child is established during assessment by social workers. Partnership between professionals from all disciplines is required to meet the needs of African refugee children affected by HIV/AIDS, working together to allay fears in a sensitive manner that acknowledges the child's cultural background and specific circumstances. Many initiatives have developed in response to the growing number of HIV/AIDS-affected African families in London. One of these is Barnados Positive Options, a scheme in which the child's cultural background is taken into account in making plans for the child's future in the event of a family disruption due to HIV and AIDS.

The case studies described in this chapter have highlighted the importance of developing culturally sensitive proxyfamilies or providing access to adult carers to support childcarers living through the progressive phases of HIV and AIDS. The naturally occurring supportive role of 'aunts' and grandmothers after the death of a mother has been discussed by Levine (1996) in the American context, and could be investigated or developed further in the UK. In the absence of local kin, the role of specifically trained 'aunties' (who tend to be culturally more appropriate than, for instance, 'uncles') from the same linguistic and cultural background as childcarers needs to be explored further. Such careworkers could act as key linkpersons between children and professionals.

In the short term, professionals need to be aware of the hidden realities of children living in such families and be able to identify and offer support to children who are providing care. Too often social work assessments of families with HIV/AIDS cases are adult-focused, with the specific problems of children remaining invisible. Professionals working with AIDS-affected children need to understand children's caring roles or the family circumstances that may put children at risk of assuming caregiving roles that impinge on their rights to childhood. Furthermore there is a need to listen to the particular voices of African children in AIDS-affected families, voices that are at times silent, but nevertheless expressive (Chinouya-Mudari, 1997). The paradoxes of childhood and parenthood should be addressed in a sensitive manner that recognizes children's cultures and rights to childhood as well as the need to 'get by'. While it is the case that parental conditions have fundamentally shaped the life-worlds of these children, the children themselves may wish to set limits on the extent of this influence. Supporting children in their caring role should enable them to meet their cultural obligations and to have some space for the preoccupations of a childhood.

Notes

1 This chapter draws on findings from the HIV and Family Life Project, a London-wide study of the impact of AIDS on family life. In particular, it examines the survival strategies used at household levels by African families, and how these strategies impact on childhood. The study is being conducted at the University of North London by Martha Chinouya-Mudari and Margaret O'Brien in collaboration with Barnados. The study is part of Martha Chinouya-Mudari's doctoral thesis and is supervised by Margaret O'Brien and Anne Phoenix.

2 The principles underpinning United Nation Conventions on the Rights of the Child, and the protection of these rights, are summed up in Article 3.1 on 'the best interests of the child'. This states: 'In all actions concerning children, whether undertaken by public or private social welfare institutions, courts of law, administrative authorities or legislative bodies, the best interests of the child shall be a primary consideration'.

3 Based on pilot work conducted as part of the HIV and Family Life Project.

References

ANKRAH, M. (1993) 'The Impact of HIV/AIDS on the family and other significant relationships: the African clan revisited', in Bor, R. and Elford, J. (eds) *The Family and HIV*. London: Cassell.

BHATT, C. (1995a) *Looking at the Epidemiology: HIV and Black Communities 1*. London: HIV Project.

BHATT, C. (1995b) *Primary and Secondary HIV Prevention Issues for African Communities: HIV and Black Communities 2*. A report of the African HIV Working Group. London: HIV Project.

BOR, R. and ELFORD, J. (eds) (1994) *The Family and HIV*. London: Cassell.

CHINOUYA-MUDARI, M. (1997) *African Children as Care-givers in Families Affected by AIDS*. London: National Children's Bureau.

DEPARTMENT OF HEALTH (1989) *Introduction to the Children Act (1989). A New Framework for the Care and Upbringing of Children*. London: HMSO.

DODGE-COLE, P. (1990) 'Health implications of war in Uganda and Sudan', *Social Science and Medicine,* **31**, 6, pp. 691–98.

IMRIE, J. and COOMBES, Y. (1995) *No Time to Waste: The Scale and Dimension of the Problem of Children Affected by HIV/AIDS in the United Kingdom*. Barkingside: Barnados.

JAMES, A. and PROUT, A. (1990) *Constructing and Reconstructing Childhood*. London: Falmer Press.

LESSER, R. (1995) *London's Children: An Analysis of 1991 Census Data*. London: National Children's Bureau.

LEVINE, C. (1996) 'Children in mourning: impact of the HIV/AIDS epidemic on mothers with AIDS and their families', in Sherr, L., Hankins, C. and Bennet, L. (eds) *AIDS as a Gender Issue*. London: Taylor & Francis.

LEWIS and MEREDITH (1988) *Daughters who Care: Daughters Caring for Mothers at Home*. London: Routledge.

MAHARAJ, K. *et al.* (1996) *An Assessment of HIV Prevention Interventions with Refugee and Asylum Seekers with Particular Reference to Refugees from the African Continent*. London: Health and Education Research Unit, Institute of Education, University of London.

NEWTON, B. and BECKER, S. (1996) *Young Carers in Southwark: The Hidden Face of Community Care*. Loughborough: Loughborough University.

O'BRIEN, M. (1994) 'Allocation of resources in households: children's perspectives', *Sociological Review,* **43**, 3, pp. 501–17.

O'BRIEN, M. and BRANNEN, J. (1996) *Children in Families: Research and Policy*. London: Falmer Press.

OFFICE FOR NATIONAL STATISTICS (ONS) (1995) *Labour Force Survey*. London: Office for National Statistics.

SAVE THE CHILDREN (1995) *Towards a Children's Agenda: New Challenges for Social Development*. London: Save the Children.

WALVIN, J. (1982) *A Child's World: A Social History of English Childhood 1800–1914*. Harmondsworth: Penguin.

UNITED NATIONS HIGH COMMISSION FOR REFUGEES (UNHCR) (1994) *The State of the World's Refugees*. Harmondsworth: Penguin.

Chapter 3

Solidarity and Stress: Gender and Local Mobilization in Tanzania and Zambia

Janet M. Bujra and Carolyn Baylies

Collective action is a kind of very concrete sociological research, a process of exploring and testing the social structure and the self.

C. Barker

Two slogans recur in the campaigning literature on HIV/AIDS in Africa: 'mobilize communities' and 'empower women'. In a context where AIDS is largely transmitted heterosexually, the vast majority of sexually active adults are potentially at risk (as well as children born of infected mothers). If all members of a local community are at risk, does this common threat constitute the grounding for united action? Attempts at mobilization soon show that local communities are differentiated, hierarchical and conflictual as often as they are harmonious sites of mutual care and compassion, while AIDS itself both unites and divides. Social fissure, along the lines of gender, generation, class, religion, ethnicity, and so on, may inhibit unity in action. The contrast here with communities of interest/identity based on sexual orientation, which have served in other parts of the world as a basis for organizing against AIDS, is profound (Pollak, 1992; Altman, 1994).

The initial focus of our own research was on women's particular vulnerability in this crisis, given their greater risk of coercive sex both within and outside marriage. Rather than assuming that women were powerless to protect themselves, we reiterated Ulin's (1992) argument that in many parts of Africa women had already developed organizational skills in networks and associations of mutual support. Anchored in their everyday struggles for survival, these associational forms might be revealed and built upon in the fight against AIDS.

Compared to community mobilization, this gendered design for action raises other issues. First, it assumes a commonality of purpose and interest among women, whereas we found that women of different generations could be at odds, even where economic or cultural differences were minimal. Equally important, instead of promoting unity, attempts to empower subordinate social categories expose and foment division. Processes of empowerment threaten to collide as women and young people assert their rights against those of a beleaguered community power structure, against men or against the older generation. A reinforcement of the solidarity and strengths of subgroupings can entrench social divisions without necessarily protecting the newly assertive.

The AIDS crisis throws these dilemmas into tragic relief. Women may question the time-honoured power and control of men, but their own safe enjoyment of sex and childbearing cannot be guaranteed without men's consent. Young people need a compact with the older generation if they are to be safer. Building bridges and transcending differences are as crucial to success as subaltern solidarity in effectively addressing the epidemic.

What follows describes the promise as well as the pitfalls of a project which included an element of action research and aimed at a level of participatory engagement. Its value rests on our initial premises about how to evaluate success, highlighted through what we call 'indicators of transformation' in AIDS work. Four such transformations are of particular significance:

1. Transformations at the level of speech, cultural expression and level of awareness about AIDS and its understanding. Such developments may breach a culture of silence about the disease (as private nightmare, as shameful disclosure, as moral degradation). They are the easiest form of change for the researcher to track, as breakthroughs in understanding or expression are recorded in everyday conversation, in interviews, focus groups or workshop transactions.
2. Transformations in behaviour around the disease itself: e.g. Collective modes of caring for the sick, supporting those who are bereaved, or arming people with knowledge about means of prevention and care. Again the observation and recording of such actions is not in itself problematic.
3. Transformations at the interpersonal level, such as greater negotiating or refusal skills in relation to sexual encounters of those who would usually have been subordinate and acquiescent partners. The researcher cannot usually access this data directly, relying instead on hearsay and assertion, which may be unreliable.
4. Structural transformations which secure, support and consolidate behavioural, cultural and interpersonal changes. There is a paradox here, for the institutionalization of innovation may stifle and contain popular creative energy. But if there is no evidence over time of greater inclusiveness and equality (e.g. in political or economic groupings and markers), then the claim that change has occurred in AIDS-related behaviour remains mere assertion. The sustainability of collective action depends to a large degree on its routinization.

Overall, we would argue that despite a background of poverty and limited resources, the major impulse to change and the effort to transform the context of risk must come from local people themselves and be under their control. Donor dependency, or what some have called the 'mendicant attitude' (Mavrocordatos and Martin, 1996: 70) limits the authenticity and sustainability of behavioural change. We do not claim that transformation of this far-reaching kind was observed or initiated in the case studies which follow, but that the points made above offer a way of assessing partial outcomes. In evaluating our work, we emphasize that interpretations might not coincide with those of members of the communities involved.

Lushoto

Lushoto is a mountainous district in the northeast of Tanzania. The research here focused on a 'village' of over 3,000 people (clustered in ten settlements) several miles from the district capital. Its people, who live by peasant farming, are predominantly Sambaa Muslims. For several generations men have left this area of high population density, land scarcity and soil erosion to seek work in urban areas. In recent decades women, and especially young women, have joined the migratory flow. Both men and women trade and sometimes find work in the nearby district capital, a 'frontier town' full of the young disaffected, gangsters, thieves, drug dealers, sex workers and strangers.

In 1995 the prevalence of HIV in the district was still relatively low for Tanzania, only 5.6 per cent among blood donors.[1] Although initially confined to those who had travelled or worked outside, the epidemic is now becoming locally entrenched. Despite these developments, limited local resources meant that virtually no AIDS work had taken place in the villages. As the epidemic began, the signs and portents of disaster were suppressed in the collective consciousness of village people; at least, they were interpreted as what happens to others – the immoral, the 'promiscuous', those greedy for money, drunkards and strangers. It was when the disease hit nearer home that people began to be afraid:

> One of my in-laws had it, and his two wives died, then his children
> and then he died.
> My sister died of it right here. She was a trader in Muheza and she
> met someone who gave it to her.

When it arrived it drew in others, forcing them to acknowledge what they would rather have denied:

> We are called to visit the sick and the dying, and to bury them.
> I heard about it at work (in the district capital) when one young man
> became infected. We all contributed money for him – Sh100 each.
> But both he and his wife died.

Still people resisted the incorporation of AIDS into their own assessment of risk:

If you are faithful you don't get it.

Not me, I respect myself.
No I'm not afraid of getting it because I understand the problem.

But it soon became clear that everyone was a potential victim, and moreover, at most risk from those to whom they were closest and needed to trust:

You are worried that your wife might have it, that she might not be faithful to you.
My husband could bring it from Dar es Salaam, so I am afraid.
My husband goes out and I don't know where he is or what he is doing.

'Extreme' forms of reaction were imagined which transgressed the normal rules of engagement between marital partners:

I will keep away from him and look after my children.
I will refuse sex with him and seek a divorce.
Send her to hospital, divorce her.
Better I live alone like a small child – not marrying, not bearing children – for the fear of this disease which has destroyed all that was sweet and pleasurable in life.

And 'extreme' forms of response were sometimes put into effect. One woman whose husband was away in Dar es Salaam received a letter informing her that her husband had AIDS. When he returned home she refused to have sex with him:

He's dead now. She's alive.

These quotations come from conversations or survey material gathered in 1995, the first year of research. They constitute confidential expressions of fear and anxiety exchanged in private. At a more public level, AIDS had also begun to figure in what could be spoken. Those who returned from urban areas had been exposed to public health messages; the few who had radios heard public health warnings even in the villages. Where talk of sexual matters had been considered shameful and a breach of respect, especially between people of adjacent generations, this was now changing. Few people considered that the new openness was a virtue; they were shocked that 'these days people can even talk about sexual matters in front of their mothers!' or they said that 'the ways of town have been brought here'. At the same time it was dawning on people that the silence of the past was a barrier to protecting their own children ('if you want them to live!'). People were talking about the issue among themselves – women to women, men to men, young people to their peers. Most people could describe the symptoms and forms of transmission.

There were differences too in the way in which gendered and generational categories viewed the crisis of AIDS. Men in positions of power were particularly prone to apportion blame and to deflect it onto anyone but themselves. When we talked to the village leaders in the initial phase of research, it was notable that several had the same diagnosis of the problem – young women were 'running away' to towns and once there falling into immoral ways; they got infected and came back home 'to count their days'. Male religious leaders saw AIDS as 'God's Big Stick' – a divine punishment visited on the sinful for their moral turpitude. And who more sinful than decadent and rebellious young people, and especially young women? Young people themselves had a different story to tell. Unmarried girls often denied any knowledge of sex or AIDS at all (cultural taboos on its acknowledgement rather than a real deficit of knowledge most probably produced this result). Among some young men there was the bravado which produced a different diagnosis of AIDS – it was unpredictable like an 'accident at work', and one could not prepare for it.

To talk about AIDS as a general issue was quite different to responding to real instances of it as a community. This was underlined by a death which took place at the end of the first phase of fieldwork. The man who died, Tourabi, had been a conductor on the buses which ply between Lushoto and Tanga on the coast (where many go seeking work). The poverty of health service provision in the area, with neither doctor nor medical assistant in the village, meant that Tourabi, like other sick people, had to be carried down steep paths to the district hospital (a one-hour walk). When the hospital sent him home the next day he was carried back. People hinted in private that he probably had AIDS (the hospital later confirmed this), but did not attend to his needs. He was living in dire straits after having been ill for months, unable to work. All his savings had gone on local medicines. He had twice married, and his second wife had borne him no children. He died the day after his return from hospital and was buried by the men of the village. The following year we asked about his wife. She had gone home to her family some distance away and no one knew whether she lived or had herself been infected and died.

Gender and Action on AIDS

There was a symmetry between men and women in terms of individual responses to AIDS, each knew that the other could kill. This had begun to generate many imagined and rather fewer actual compromises with patriarchy. But for most the reality was more like that of Tourabi's wife. A wife may suspect her husband is sick but he denies it or even threatens her, and she is unable to refuse him sexual relations. When she is widowed, others may suspect her of having infected him; and as a woman, her rights to continued use of his land to satisfy subsistence needs are dependent on her having borne children. As Tourabi's wife had borne no child, she was left destitute.

This is a community in which men and women are far from equal. Men of the same patrilineage live together all their lives while wives marry in as strangers. They are responsible for most of the agricultural work required to feed their families, even though the land they work never becomes theirs. Women do not inherit land, but they might hold it in trust for their sons. All the key positions of political and religious leadership are taken by men. Men consider themselves to have rights over the bodies of their wives, rights for sex, for procreation and for beating ('if she has done wrong'). Despite this, women here could be said to form a 'submerged network', 'achieving sometimes via informal activities of everyday resistance a partial penetration of authority's claims' (Barker 1997: 7). Perhaps precisely because women could not call on each other as kinsfolk, although needing each other in times of childbirth, hardship and harvest, they had over the generations continually recreated a network of mutual support known as *kidembwa*.

This network (it had no overall direction or centralized leadership) consisted of the cohort of older women, those who had already borne children, and who acted as midwives and as honorary grandparents to socialize young people, especially girls. They were capable, through the network, of amassing large amounts of money for disbursement when their sons got married and at the birth of their first grandchild. The institution of *kidembwa* was submerged because it had no obvious presence or representation in the formal political and religious life of the village. Indeed, it was sometimes hostile to this male-dominated hierarchy. When funds were disbursed, the elderly women brewed beer. Women became intoxicated in a celebration from which *men were excluded. The subversive nature of this in a Muslim setting is unsettling, and the *kidembwa* was viewed with distaste and dismissal by many men.

While subversive in one sense, exclusive to women and protective of women's secret knowledge of childbirth, the *kidembwa* women were also complicit in upholding patriarchal power. In marriage ceremonies they initiated young women into the secrets of sex and giving pleasure to husbands, and it was they who upheld the prescription of virginity in brides by celebrating those who were intact on marriage and exposing those who were not. How could such a powerful but submerged and subversive network be sparked into collective action on the issue of AIDS? The action component of this research was devoted to finding ways to build on the existing pattern of social relations in order to borrow strength and a promise of sustainability in a collective struggle against AIDS, but without simply resurrecting the terms of women's existing oppression, especially young women's.

The Process

The aims were both practical and ambitious, based on the knowledge gained in the first phase of research. The first was to question the culture of silence over AIDS in the village so that it could be embraced as a collective responsibility. The second was to build bridges to link village people with medical personnel in the district hospital so they could get more help, and to bridge social categories of gender and generation in the village to offer a context in which differences could be publicly and safely aired and some movement towards positive resolution achieved.

This was attempted through the following activities. A series of workshops were held in different settlements of the village, facilitated by AIDS activists from the capital who were involved in our project. By providing transport we were also able to involve the hospital AIDS coordinating officer and the newly appointed AIDS counsellor. The workshops, separate for men and women, were attended by upwards of 250 people. At the conclusion of each workshop, two representatives were chosen, one older and one younger, to coordinate efforts for the whole community. At the same time, a group for young women was formed out of the cohort of school girls who had left the local primary school in 1995. These girls were keen to find ways of earning an income which did not entail them leaving for the towns. Through our efforts the young women began to be taught machine sewing and were granted a piece of land by the village chairman. They arranged a celebratory opening for the group to which everyone in the village was invited, and despite three funerals having taken place that day, it attracted a large audience, including village political and religious leaders and invited guests from the district capital. They prepared songs and put on a small play about AIDS.[2] The same group put on a second performance for girls at the local school with the intention of drawing their next set of members from the departing cohort of 1996. A few days later, all the village representatives (12, with men and women, young and old in equal proportions) came together to discuss what they could do next and made plans for how they would work. This group of coordinators agreed to befriend and care for those who were sick and to maintain an awareness about risk among all people, but especially the young.

There are several obvious achievements of this phase of collective action. Firstly, the culture of silence around AIDS was well and truly breached, perhaps for ever. This was not simply a matter of 'education', though our workshops had entailed the imparting of knowledge about the transmission of HIV, the signs of AIDS, forms of protection, and what could be done to help those infected. It was more that the subject had been put on the community agenda in a non-judgemental way, with an emphasis on truth, openness and caring. AIDS had begun to be seen as everyone's responsibility.

Secondly, hospital staff were able to convey that they were willing and ready to help local people in a limited way, so reducing the antipathy people had initially felt against the hospital which 'sent people home to die'. Thirdly, distant settlements which were normally not reached by outsiders had been brought into the process and had participated on an impressive scale. Fourthly, women had spoken openly of their fears and perceptions of men as the most blameworthy in this epidemic. They had been drawn into the action through the network of the *kidembwa* (all the older women chosen as representatives were elders in that institution). Fifthly, the invisibility of young women had been diminished and they had found a way of increasing their stature in the eyes of village leaders through their new association. Finally, for men and women to discuss matters of sexuality together on equal terms, as they did in our final meeting, was something previously unheard of. Through this work, issues of gender inequity came to the fore, they were 'resolved' at the level of discourse and people made plans together so they could face the crisis of AIDS.

It is worth noting some key moments in the process of change, where conflict and contradiction were revealed in discourse and action. The first came from a woman's workshop attended by some of the more prominent elders in the *kidembwa* network. What was revealing about this encounter was that it displayed a rehearsal of challenges to men's control of sexuality so that women might protect themselves. An older woman spontaneously imagined what she might say to her husband returning from Dar es Salaam, 'All right husband, you are home and let's celebrate, but use that condom! And if you haven't got one, then I'll go and sleep elsewhere! Or if you keep forgetting, then buy them for me to keep!' Other women were howling with laughter and shame at her frankness, covering their faces with their wrappers. An old woman intervened, 'Some men get drunk and they refuse to use these things and they can beat you!' But the first responded with bravado, 'Yes! It's true. He will beat you but at least you have told him plainly! Better to be beaten than to die!'

At the same time, this workshop disclosed the hostility of older women towards the young, and of many towards people with AIDS. A young woman asked daringly, 'Aren't there any condoms for women?' Whereupon the older women turned round and glared: 'Who said that? You young women are too much! You want it [sex] too badly. . . . People will say you are a prostitute!' Later, when the facilitator asked how people with AIDS could be cared for and described their needs and the risks of attending to them, someone burst out, 'Isn't that why we avoid people with this disease? People put them near to the lavatory, away from all the others in the house.'

A meeting held with some of the *kidembwa* elders a few weeks after the workshops revealed their struggles with dangerous dilemmas. As midwives, where contact with blood could put them at risk of infection, they determined to find ways to purchase rubber gloves. What about taking care of those who were actually ill? For the first time we heard people name those believed to be afflicted; there were more men who had the signs than women, but their wives were in danger. Hesitantly they suggested talking to the women, and getting older men to befriend the men in question and offer help. The breakthrough was their acknowledgement that men and women would have to act together if productive action was to be taken.

In the final meeting of village representatives there were other break-throughs. A discussion of AIDS led, with little prompting, to a questioning of the gendered division of labour in the domestic arena. When one man blamed mothers for young people's immoral behaviour, the women were incensed. The confrontation was resolved, however, by two men taking the women's side and acknowledging that men had to change. They did not support their wives in bringing up the children, 'We give orders, we are dictators in our homes.'

There was also a significant shift in generational relations at this same meeting. The younger women acted as spokespersons for older women who were uneasy and inhibited in a totally novel setting. And the *kidembwa* women as a whole gave their backing to the girls' group, and began to work out moves to extend their traditional role as mentors in raising awareness of AIDS issues among the young.

By the following year (1997) it was possible to see the extent to which the promise of the work was being delivered. The most successful initiative had been the girls' group, as they secured funding for a brickmaking project from an external donor. Unfortunately, this set them at odds with young men jealously challenging gender differences. The *kidembwa* women had seen the value of external help and were trying to set up a bank account so they too could apply for funding. Another man had died of AIDS, and while his wife was supported by some in the village group, she was refused a test result at the hospital through lack of funds. Two years of drought had sapped communal energy and the coordinators' group was meeting only fitfully. Whether a group founded on the equality of men and women in the fight against AIDS can be sustained and effective when it transgresses all the usual gendered arrangements remains to be seen. What happens at the most public level does not necessarily translate into transformation at the most intimate level, and in the end only this will allow for greater safety in the struggle against AIDS.

Mansa

Research conducted in Zambia confirmed our original hypothesis: it is possible to harness women's existing organizational skills, grounded in networks of mutual support, for campaigns of protection against AIDS. But it also highlighted potential obstacles to effective mobilization. The study site reported on here was a set of peri-urban villages on the outskirts of Mansa, the provincial headquarters for Luapula Province. Predominantly Christian and Bemba-speaking, some residents are locally born, but others come from different locations within the province as well as from other parts of Zambia. While sharing many cultural commonalities, including similar patterns of gender relations, the community is less homogeneous than in Lushoto. Their heterogeneity also applied to their economic circumstances, which range from government employment and successful commerce to severe poverty, with meagre if any reliable income.

HIV prevalence in Mansa is higher than in Lushoto, with 23 per cent of women attending antenatal clinics at the local hospital affected (1994). Limited testing facilities and a disinclination of most to have tests means than there is considerable uncertainty about the cause of the deaths which occur with such frequency. But, at the same time, familiarity with the symptoms of AIDS leads many to 'know' of its presence in their own and others' homes. Survey data showed that, compared with Lushoto (45%), a considerably higher proportion of those in Mansa (77%) were personally acquainted with or related to someone who had AIDS:

> Most of the people whom I used to know have passed away.
> I have seen them suffering.
> I know many who have died.
> Three of my fellow teachers have died.
> I myself have AIDS.

People were generally knowledgeable about means of protection; many felt they were heeding warnings and therefore might be safe:

> I cannot be infected because I avoid casual sex.
> I try very much to avoid sex before marriage.
> I know all about the disease and how to protect myself.

Others, however, expressed self-doubt and worries about partners who might not be faithful:

> If I am not careful . . .
> If the condom is not used during sex . . .
> Maybe your partner can be infected from somewhere else and then infect you later.

Previous Initiatives

Unlike rural Lushoto, Mansa had been the site of numerous AIDS initiatives with both state and external donor involvement and funding. A scheme under the United Nations Development Programme (UNDP) had been in place for a number of years headed by an international coordinator working with local volunteers. One initiative under this scheme was the setting up of a teen centre to foster health education and provide recreational facilities for unemployed young people in the town. A government programme to train community-based AIDS workers and to support a team delivering pre- and post-test hospital counselling, follow-up at clinics and home-based care was begun in 1992. Anti-AIDS clubs were in place in many of the schools.

Despite this level of input, efforts and activities remain truncated, episodic and incomplete, their potential unfulfilled. By 1995 the pre-test hospital counselling programme was operating unevenly either through lack of test kits or the non-availability of counsellors. The home-based care programme had run into difficulties through lack of coordination and insufficient transport. The work of the anti-AIDS club at a local primary school was temporarily suspended as staff and students gave their energies to the digging of a well. Plans to assist orphans had foundered on lack of funds after initially hopeful discussions with local church officials. Only one of those trained as a community AIDS worker was still conducting AIDS education, glossed with a distinctively Christian call for fidelity.

A problem encountered throughout involved resourcing voluntary efforts, given the level of poverty in the area. Because some early AIDS initiatives supported by donors incorporated allowances for local participants, an expectation had been nurtured among some that compensation should be forthcoming for community work. When allowances dried up, all too frequently the 'voluntary work' dried up as well. One of the elders, who had also received training as a community AIDS worker, related how anti-AIDS efforts dwindled and then ceased altogether because no allowances were given and squabbles arose over who should have access to bicycles which had been made available to them. This man baulked at the suggestion that the group might be reassembled, saying there was little sense in trying to do so unless allowances were to be offered. As the research proceeded, it became clear we could not simply assume that previous groundwork provided a basis on which renewed activity might be based, or harbour the illusion that our presence would serve as a catalyst for a phoenix-like regeneration of activities or consolidation of effort, even though this seemed to be an unspoken hope of officials in district and provincial officers assigned to AIDS work. Rather, the reasons for past problems had to be confronted.

Collective Responses

The pattern of frequently frustrated enthusiasm and recurrent problems of sustainability both provided the context for our research and added urgency to the need to identify modes of intervention and forms of organization that 'worked'. While attempting to assess the causes of impeded success in the past, we also monitored several new initiatives. Following a series of focus group discussions, three groups were identified which seemed to have the capacity for voluntary action. The Muchinka Women's Drama Group was formed by a number of women who ran stalls in the local Muchinka market. Members of the Natweshe Women's Club were drawn from a village on the outskirts of Mansa. Street Kids was a donor-funded project set up to develop skills among Mansa's school-leavers. Whereas the drama group had an exclusive AIDS focus, the other two hoped to add AIDS work to their organization's existing income-generating activities.

Further discussions were initiated with these groups about AIDS and what they might do to protect themselves and others. The research team also observed the groups' activities and served as a bridge between them and those at district and provincial level charged with coordinating AIDS activities. Our objective was to clarify the strengths and weaknesses of collective efforts so as to identify factors influencing the sustainability and effectiveness of AIDS work at the level of the community. At the same time, we wanted to assess the impact of this collective work on the participants themselves and to explore their engagement with issues of gender.

The Muchinka Women's Drama Group

The eight women in the Muchinka Women's Drama Group were in their thirties and forties, all married, with an average of four children each. All were market traders, and their AIDS drama group was built on an existing network of shared interests and mutual economic assistance. They drew inspiration and commitment from their experiences as mothers and wives, with responsibilities straddling the domestic sphere and the external generation of income. One among them had been involved in a drama group active several years earlier in another part of the province, Kashikashi, as part of a donor-sponsored AIDS initiative. Participants in that case had received an allowance when they performed. The Muchinka market women reworked the scripts which had been used in Kashikashi, embellishing them with their own ideas.

Within a few months they had prepared two 20-minute presentations. One portrayed a mother encouraging her daughter to marry a rich suitor so as to lift the family from its state of poverty. The strategy ended in tragedy when the daughter subsequently became ill and died, whereupon her younger sister was inherited by the husband and, in turn, succumbed to AIDS. The tale was a cautionary one, reflecting suspicions directed at older, wealthy males seeking young women as sexual partners, and subjecting to scrutiny customs such as widow inheritance which, in the era of AIDS, can be a source of particular danger. The women performed their plays at the local health clinic to responsive, predominantly female audiences. Their enthusiasm and effectiveness particularly impressed a visiting UNDP delegation in the summer of 1996, to whom they were held up as a model of local initiative.

When asked during a further discussion to reflect on why they had set up their group, they readily replied, 'To educate ourselves and others.' They found it more difficult to assess the group's benefit to them on a personal level since, as they explained, these matters were difficult to speak of openly. 'We try to teach our husbands,' they said. One added, 'It could be that I am aware of it and the husband is reluctant to understand this.' Another said, 'The only problem lies with the men. Women understand better than men.' Their solution was that 'men as well should be invited to their own offices for their lesson'.

Group members were committed and able, but also aware of the costs incurred in this community work. When rehearsing and performing they had to leave their market stalls, and the impact of the lost income was keenly felt. They argued that some compensation or material assistance was required if they were to continue giving their performances. They would be more effective, they said, if they could afford the semblance of a 'uniform' – a T-shirt or wrappers displaying the name of their group – and if they distributed condoms after presenting their plays. Quite understandably they endeavoured to use the research team as a conduit to those with resources, and we accepted the function of liaising as a legitimate aspect of our research task. Although reasserting their commitment to continue with their work, fewer performances were given in subsequent months and the issue of resourcing remained a sore one.

Natweshe Women's Club

The second group whose progress we observed was the Natweshe Women's Club, set up in September 1995 to enhance income-generating activities, but foundering shortly thereafter. A focus group discussion held on AIDS in the village in April 1996 revived enthusiasm among the women to reorganize their group and, moreover, to include AIDS education among their objectives. By the end of May 1996 the group had 18 registered members, all from the village and all married women. They came together as neighbours and as women in similar economic circumstances and family situations. From the beginning most of their husbands were strongly supportive of their activities, which were seen as making a material contribution to individual families. They aimed to raise a small amount of capital through membership fees and use it as seed money for a collective activity, perhaps a garden or tailoring. One woman who had been trained in knitting by the Catholic Church began to teach this skill to several of her fellow members.

Further discussion with members of the research team on matters of AIDS prevention led them to conclude that they should involve men. While some expressed scepticism, they proposed to invite their husbands to a subsequent meeting. A 'couples meeting' was arranged and participants were encouraged to attend via personal visits from one of the most active members and her husband. Although numbers were small, the initiative was promising, allowing opportunity for husbands and wives to speak in one another's company with unusual openness.

When the research team met with the Natweshe women in August 1996, the occasion was a poignant one. The husband of the most active woman had just died, a reminder to all – though little did they need it – of the immediacy of the threat of AIDS. However, the women also explained proudly that they had now initiated a brickmaking project to construct a meeting place. Many of their husbands were working with them and a number attended the meeting. One man said by way of explaining his presence, 'I thought that only women come here, but I came to know later, when my wife told me, that even we were wanted.'

In reporting back to them the findings of the earlier stage of our research, further discussion ensued regarding AIDS and the use of condoms. This raised the question of gender relations which, in the past (and perhaps in some cases in the present) had condoned the beating of wives. The forum provided opportunity for bringing into the open behaviour seldom subject to public scrutiny or critical comment, the presence of husbands permitting words to be spoken and heard which individual couples might feel unable to speak directly to one another.

Street Kids

The Street Kids group consisted of both males and females who had been forced, through lack of funds, to drop out of school. Many lived not just in poor conditions but in disrupted family circumstances, with a single parent or with another relative. They had been brought together via an externally deter-mined agenda (and source of funds) rather than on the basis of their own initiative. Although they now worked collectively, cultivating a vegetable plot and raising chickens, the group's history and nature were quite different from those of the Muchinka Women's Drama Group or the Natweshe Women's Club.

An initial focus group discussion about AIDS was held with several of the male members of the Street Kids, with a subsequent session, involving both males and females, held to discuss ways in which they might work together on AIDS. Members of the group suggested that they might become peer educa-tors, with girls talking to girls and boys to boys. They knew many who were engaged in selling sexual favours or otherwise putting themselves at risk. Several further meetings were arranged to finalize plans, but the researchers found themselves waiting in vain for the group to turn up. Individuals pro-fessed willingness to proceed, but collective action proved elusive.

Comparative Assessment of the Three Groups

Working with the groups suggested that their relative success in achieving objectives and promoting AIDS awareness (as well as confronting the gender issues invariably thrown up in the process), varied according to the positioning of AIDS work within their broader concerns. It also varied with the composi-tion of the groups and of their target audiences and in response to the issue of resourcing efforts or calculating benefits. What seemed to emerge from an initial evaluation of the three groups was that AIDS work is most effective when well focused, based on perceived needs and solidly grounded in the common interests of those involved in a collective endeavour.

The exclusive focus of the Muchinka drama group on AIDS education and prevention seemed to have been a feature of strength, and some members' enthusiasm for an enlarged agenda was a cause of concern lest this dilute its effectiveness. At the same time, the progress made by the Natweshe Women's Club on AIDS work may have been partly facilitated by the fact that work around AIDS was *not* the main reason for the group's existence, but an addition to their income-generating activities which could be activated periodically in accord with the group's development and expressed need. AIDS work can be grafted onto the activities of an existing group, but how far this proves successful depends on the history of the group, the nature of its original objectives and the extent to which the same degree of commonality informing original objectives can extend to AIDS work. That adding on AIDS activities can prove problematic is evidenced by the Street Kids' abortive proposals to engage in peer education. Here an initial concern with income generation retained an overarching importance for group members, who found it difficult to move into other areas.

The Muchinka Women's Drama Group was organized around their common concern as women with the threat posed by AIDS. But it was their existing organizational capacity – their previous networking, grounded in shared economic pursuits – which particularly facilitated their coming together to do work around AIDS. While the Street Kids seemed to share with the drama group a pattern of solidarity on the basis of shared economic activities, the youth group had a more artificial solidarity, given their recruitment as individuals and the goal of their organization to foster the individual acquisition of skills. Moreover, although similar in age, the Street Kids did not belong to so clearly bounded a constituency as did the Muchinka women. When asked what they might do about AIDS, the Street Kids helpfully suggested peer education. But this proved a difficult endeavour to take on, especially given proposed reliance on individual initiative and oriented toward a large and rather ill-defined target group.

The Natweshe Club had a clearly bounded constituency based on common residence, if initially only a vague sense of what they might do as regards AIDS, save that they should themselves be the targets of any activity. As they began to discuss AIDS, they soon resolved that any effective action must involve inclusion of their husbands. This was an important recognition and instructive as regards our own research. While utilizing women's organizational capacities, the process of collective action and reflection led quickly to a recognition of the need to embrace potentially conflicting interests in order to ensure a broader sense of community and a more secure, mutual protection. The drama group also conceded the need for men to be brought in to AIDS education efforts. Having defined their own efforts as directed at women, however, they suggested not that they do this themselves but that a parallel effort should be undertaken by a male group. The fact that the Street Kids included both males and females at the outset might have proved beneficial in allowing a forum across gender lines, yet because it was never closely confronted as an issue, gender may have served more to divide than to bring the group together over the issue of AIDS.

The individualistic orientation of the Street Kids raises the question of the extent to which initiatives around AIDS are successfully able to combine personal interest with the broader community welfare. A source of strength of the Muchinka women was their homogeneity with respect to their gender, their economic pursuits and their marital status. But if describing a common vulnerability to AIDS, this basis of recruitment also brought to the fore their worries about the way in which 'community work' potentially interfered with their individual livelihood strategies. Although some progress was being made, it was not always easy for members to square an equation relating personal economic cost to community health benefits. In contrast, the fact that the Natweshe women (and their husbands) were more explicitly their own target group meant that the link between altruistic community activity and self/collective interest was a solid one, and at least in this regard the question of compensation did not immediately present itself.

Conclusions

The material we have discussed here underlines the need to eschew unthinking notions of 'community mobilization'. The 'community's' own internal complexities and divisions are always on the agenda in any process of transformation; indeed, they are exposed by any bid to empower previously subordinate social categories. Our focus here was on the way in which such divisions may be creatively exploited in the struggle against AIDS. In Lushoto we looked at a local community where there had been no previous AIDS initiatives and where the aim was to generate a community response which bridged the divisions of gender and generation while still addressing women's particular vulnerabilities. In Mansa, women were beginning to organize themselves for active involvement in AIDS initiatives, or were stimulated to do so by the research project itself, and the aim here was to assess and support these efforts as well as to gain further understanding of why in some cases they had not worked or been sustained. An important concern in each case was the extent to which such initiatives could transcend their gendered origins, bringing men on board.

Both these cases show the value of, and the difficulties in, drawing on women's existing organizational capacities in the fight against AIDS. Women are not only more vulnerable to infection; they often have closer ties of mutuality than men, founded in their greater economic insecurity and their need for assistance at times of life crises. These life crises are themselves highly relevant to the transmission of AIDS, focusing as they do on birth and sex. In some cases women's associational talents are already fully employed; in other cases they are invisible, repressed and unremarked, and a spark may be required to ignite them into action.

Our research also underlines the point that it is not enough for women to mobilize. The question is whether and how men can be brought into a struggle, which in so far as it demands greater mutuality between the sexes, also means that those who presently have greater power now have more to lose. Men have less incentive to change; their own vulnerabilities can be addressed by even harsher patriarchal measures: regimes of surveillance on wives, girlfriends, daughters or sisters, or the seeking out of virgin girls; they can abandon suspected partners more easily than women can afford to be abandoned. Men, moreover, can *choose* to use condoms whereas women can only choose to be celibate. Only at two points are men more vulnerable: they may need woman-care if they fall sick and they too need to have unprotected sex if they are to bear children. All of these points need to be considered further in any strategy for building alliances across gender lines.

In both Lushoto and Mansa a sea change had occurred at the discursive level. People had begun to organize themselves for caring and awareness-raising in relation to AIDS. They were still rehearsing interpersonal change, while structural transformation was limited. Self-reliance in resourcing voluntary effort was stretching some people beyond the bounds of altruism.

Finally, this study carries the message that AIDS work cannot be advanced in a day, precisely because it demands social transformations rather than rapid technological fixes or individual acts of enlightenment. As compared to the short-termism of many AIDS interventions, the method we have described here involves the long-term mapping out and enhancement of qualitative change, the ultimate outcomes of which cannot be predicted.

Acknowledgements

The research reported on here was funded by the ESRC (R00235221). It involved teamworking at six sites: Dar es Salaam, Lushoto and Mbeya in Tanzania and Lusaka, Mansa and Mongu in Zambia. The work of Julius Mwabuki and Naomi Kaihula in Lushoto and Arnold Kunda and Tashisho Chabala in Mansa requires special acknowledgement. For the theoretical grounding of the project see Baylies and Bujra (1995).

Notes

1 The estimates are based on a biased sample as blood donors are drawn almost exclusively from the healthy male kin of a sick person, a category which may well have high seropositivity compared to the population as a whole.

2 The play was a somewhat didactic piece about a young girl returning from Dar es Salaam infected with HIV. It included 'warnings' about the dangers to young women (but not young men) of leaving for a life in town; more positively it took up the challenge from the workshops about breaking the culture of silence and avoidance of AIDS patients and contained strong messages about 'living positively' with AIDS.

References

ALTMAN, D. (1994) *Power and Community: Organisational and Cultural Responses to AIDS*. London: Taylor & Francis.

BARKER, C. (1997) 'Empowerment and resistance: "Collective Effervescence" and other accounts'. Paper presented to the Annual Conference of the British Sociological Association, York, April.

BAYLIES, C. and BUJRA, J. (1995) 'Discourses of power and empowerment in the fight against HIV/AIDS in Africa', in Aggleton, P. *et al.* (eds) *AIDS: Safety, Sexuality and Risk*. London: Taylor & Francis.

MAVROCORDATOS, A. and MARTIN, P. (1995) 'Theatre for development: listening to the community', in Nelson, N. and Wright, S. (eds) *Power and Participatory Development*. London: Intermediate Technology Publications.

POLLAK, M. (1992) *AIDS: A Problem for Sociological Research*. London: Sage.

ULIN, P. (1992) 'African women and AIDS: negotiating behavioural change', *Social Science and Medicine*, **34**, 1, pp. 63–73.

Chapter 4

Gender, Disclosure, Care and Decision Making in KwaZulu-Natal, South Africa: A Pilot Programme using Storytelling Techniques

Gill Seidel and Rosalind Coleman

An exploratory study on gender, decision making and the disclosure of HIV serostatus was carried out in Hlabisa in rural KwaZulu-Natal in South Africa in 1995. This chapter describes the context in which the work was conducted and the interactive and problem-solving storytelling techniques that were used to access sensitive information. Linear and didactic story forms that were already being used by peer group educators in the region were adapted in order to gather new data about the dynamics of disclosure, and in order to 'envoice' rural people, particularly women.

Hlabisa district has a population of approximately 205,000 people. Once part of Zululand, now KwaZulu-Natal (KWZ), and situated in largely tribal trust land, the vast majority of its people are Zulu-speakers. Most live in scattered rural homesteads, but there is also one urban area, and one small informal settlement. There is widespread malnutrition. With mere subsistence farming, the main sources of income are pension remittances and income from migrant labour outside the area. According to 1994 statistics from the Development Bank of Southern Africa, the literacy rate in the region is 69% and life expectancy is 63 years. Government health services are provided by a 300-bed district hospital, 10 satellite village clinics, and a mobile clinic service. The clinics are staffed by nurses, and a doctor visits each of the village clinics once a month, but does not travel with the mobile service. There is one non-governmental organization (NGO) in the district, specializing in community development. Between 1992 and 1997, the HIV prevalence in women attending antenatal clinic in Hlabisa district was rising rapidly (Figures 4.1 and 4.2).

The need for care and support is beyond what can be met through existing government and NGO services. And these services cannot be guaranteed in the community, not only because of the possible rejection of the HIV positive people by their families and household members, but also because women are infected at a younger age than men. They are therefore less likely to be able to perform their 'traditional' caring role (Heise and Elias, 1995) in circumstances

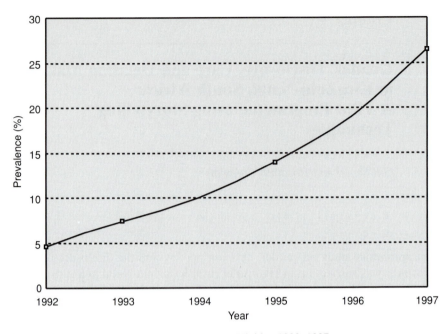

Figure 4.1   Antenatal HIV seroprevalence, Hlabisa 1992–1997.

where such interpretations of normative practices and understandings are also political definitions in that they can be contested, and have material consequences (Moore, 1994).

A group of HIV positive people began to meet together in 1994. As they discussed their future needs, it became apparent that one of their major concerns was the issue of disclosing HIV status at home. Safe disclosure was only possible where the recipient of the information was well informed about HIV and AIDS and accepting of HIV positive people. It was in this context that the study described here was undertaken. The work coincided with an ongoing programme of training and education of HIV positive and lay people, as well as traditional healers, who are known to play a key role in determining community behaviour patterns (Coleman, 1996). Wider aspects of the work relating to confidentiality, disclosure and support, and different urban and rural emphases in South Africa, are discussed elsewhere (Seidel, 1996b).

The Genesis of the Project

The project was conceived in March 1994 during a workshop on developing a KwaZulu home-based care programme for people with HIV/AIDS. The main findings from a local participatory evaluation were being presented and dis-

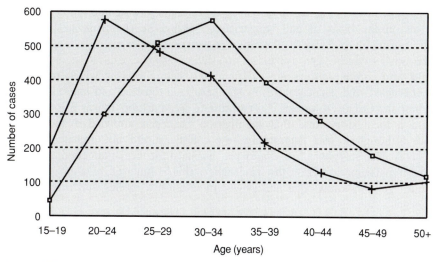

Figure 4.2 Age–sex distribution of reported AIDS cases in South Africa 1994: (□) male, (+) female.

cussed (Soldan, Abdool-Karim and Abdool-Karim, 1994; Ross, Nxumalo and Philpott, 1994). The principal recommendation to arise from the workshop was that counsellors should place greater emphasis in pre- and post-test counselling on the importance of naming a caregiver within the family. There were persuasive public health reasons for this decision. Above all, it would facilitate the work of hard-pressed nurses. Because of the code of confidentiality for HIV adhered to locally, nurses involved in home-based care were not able to educate the family about HIV, and the practical measures to adopt when caring for a seropositive family member. This main recommendation was received pragmatically, and altogether uncontroversially.

But what of the gender dynamics? There are a number of issues to be considered here, especially in view of the fact that young women are by far the most affected, most probably because young women have their first sexual experiences with older men and, according to many largely informal accounts, this is rarely consensual sex (Armstrong, 1994; Wood, Maforah and Jewkes, 1996). In this context, and with a desire to make any intervention gender-sensitive rather than add to the burden of women's unpaid work, these initial concerns formed the basis for the identification of a number of more formal hypotheses. Central among these were: What is the gender of the caregiver and care receiver? Who cares for whom, and more specifically, who cares for women who are HIV symptomatic? Additionally, what is the status of the largely informal data – important gendered information that often eludes formal studies – which suggests that women who disclose their serostatus to their partner face violence, rejection and homelessness? (Temmerman *et al.*, 1995; Rotherberg and Paskey, 1995).

Much prevailing health discourse is not gender aware and tends to generalize on the basis of male experience, taking the (heterosexual) man as the norm. In so doing, it glosses over women's experience. Indeed, one of the small group of persons with HIV/AIDS who participated in the workshop, and who courageously shared their experience, a sharing which minimizes 'otherness', told participants how she had been rejected and made homeless when she disclosed her HIV serostatus to her partner. It was a local voice and a local story, one that highlighted gendered knowledge and abuse; but although it was listened to respectfully, it did not appear to carry weight. Her story was heard and yet 'unheard'; it went unheeded, implying token participation. For the researcher, this stimulated existing concerns about gender, knowledge and power in relation to policy and intervention designs.

More detailed enquiry into the decision-making processes surrounding disclosure patterns for different women and men (in relation to HIV, TB and STDs since these are interrelated), their outcomes, and the support networks available, seemed both legitimate and necessary. Such a project would involve eliciting highly sensitive information via individual interviews (because of confidentiality) about social and reciprocal relations and dynamics within the family and neighbourhood. How this could be done ethically, respecting confidentiality and access, with local accountability in a limited managerial time frame and with a limited budget were issues that needed to be addressed.

The first priority was to conceptualize the problem in terms of gender and social relations, *not* in terms of a biomedical agenda (Raynaut, 1996). After that, and only then, could methodologies and a project design be considered. The broader research questions were these: (i) What are the discourses that construct gender and what are their effects locally? (ii) Through what agencies, in what conditions, and on what timescales can more sensitive agendas be introduced to question dominant constructions of gender, and to access or extend gendered rights discourse in a participatory fashion?

Storytelling: The Functions of Narratives

Narrative and storytelling would seem to be a universal phenomenon, although not everyone's story is, or has been, seen as equally legitimate (Hymes, 1996). Forms of storytelling have been used in a variety of contexts in South Africa, including in the Truth and Reconciliation Commission, to elicit very painful experiences and to generate and confront different kinds of knowledge, memory and identity. This has not only been done in the conventional anthropological sense of seeking only 'traditional' narrators and themes, but also from a more creative rights perspective in which data has applications for literacy and for policy making. Importantly, the most dynamic examples of storytelling used as part of gender and AIDS education in post-apartheid South Africa are *interactive*, with there being no single authoritative voice (Seidel, 1995). This was the model used here, and the aim was to try and work creatively within this emergent and plural practice, informed by a range of theoretical frameworks (Bakhtin, 1981; Boal, 1995; Hyden, 1997).

Illness narratives have a range of different functions (Frank, 1995). Narratives about AIDS appear distinct in that they are largely concerned with finding an opportunity to engage with a range of imagined possible scenarios. Although little research has been conducted into interactive work of this kind, and even less in a rural development context, this kind of enquiry is relevant to the problem-solving approach adopted in the study design.

The study design was influenced by stories that associations of people with HIV/AIDS in the region, assisted by health professionals, were already telling in a variety of venues, as part of community education about AIDS (Seidel, 1996a). However, these Positive Speakers' 'stories' tended to be linear, didactic, and non-participatory, other than for questions at the end. They had a fairly set pattern, which may have been shaped in part by medical history-taking and forms of counselling. They often took the following form:

- Here I am; this is my life.
- I am a person who has HIV.
- This is how I think I contracted HIV.
- This is how I felt when I knew.
- This is how some other people behaved towards me.
- This is how I live my life now.
- These are the arrangements I have made for my children.
- And this is what *you* need to know and do to avoid getting infected.

Narratives of this kind influenced our desire as part of the research design to elicit 'thicker' biographies (Bakhtin, 1981).

Eligibility Criteria and Ethics

The selection criteria for interviewees was that all had been diagnosed as HIV positive, had received pre- and post-test counselling, and had agreed through their nurse-counsellor to participate in the study. In order to respect confidentiality, access was negotiated exclusively through the counsellor. Because of this, the number of respondents was limited, a problem complicated by the fact that many nurse-counsellors were already engaged in other duties, and often had to travel considerable distances between rural homesteads. These are real constraints but they are often unfamiliar to researchers focusing conventionally on 'captive populations' (e.g. hospital patients, STD clinic attenders).

Interactive Narrative Design

In order to elicit more interactive kinds of knowledge and understanding, two 'vignettes' were constructed using available information about disclosure, outcomes, attitudes to the gender of carer, and the support networks, if any, that are available differentially to women and men. These sketches were neither factual nor fictional, but were general enough to invite identification,[1] while respecting confidentiality.

The first, *Zanile's Story*, was about a woman who is diagnosed as HIV seropositive when she attends the antenatal clinic, and the counsellor then asks her to disclose this fact to someone at home. The second, *Joseph and Thandi's Story*, focuses on Joseph, a migrant worker, diagnosed as HIV positive and with tuberculosis (TB), who had visited a traditional healer and a clinic in the past for sexually transmitted diseases (STDs), and who is now returning home to his wife in the village. Each story is deliberately unfinished.

Questions were asked in the third person to elicit the experience, situated knowledge, and insights of the interviewee. Who do you think Zanile would tell about her HIV result? Why this person, and not that one? What about her mother? Her mother-in-law? Would the mother-in-law look after Zanile? What would she think about her daughter-in-law? Why do you say that? What about her little girl at school? How would this affect her? And the boy? Similar questions designed along gendered parameters were put about Joseph and his village wife Thandi. Interviewees were also asked about HIV, STDs and TB, and about the relationship and gender of the likely carers. The final question for both stories involved asking about what might be the best possible ending under the circumstances.

Later we moved from third-person discussions about Zanile, Joseph and their imagined decision processes and outcomes, to engage the respondents who had disclosed their own HIV serostatus. Questions were asked to elicit their own experiences of disclosure, the reactions of those in the know, how these reactions/behaviours affected them, their experience(s) of care, the sources of different kinds of support at different times, perceptions of the quality or appropriateness of this care and support, and how this corresponded to their needs.

The two stories were recounted in accessible Zulu by a cofieldworker, and questions put to eight women and seven men in locations close to their home. Women in particular were very forthcoming, and many welcomed the opportunity to unburden themselves. We asked interviewees if they knew of people who had been rejected or beaten after disclosing their HIV serostatus. We also asked if respondents thought that meeting other people like them (including a peer support group) would be a good or bad idea, and why.

Findings

The gender of care being expressed largely in biological and reproductive terms, a woman was seen to be a 'natural carer' by both women and most men. As one respondent described it, '[A woman] has borne children. She knows what pain/suffering is.' It follows then that all men, single or married, can anticipate receiving care from their mother primarily, but also from wives and/ or girlfriends. There were, however, different disclosure configurations for HIV, STDs and TB (Seidel and Ntuli, 1996) with TB being the easiest condition to disclose since it is not so heavily stigmatized and is seen as being treatable.

Women interviewed tended to be relatively isolated as a result of patrilocal marriage arrangements, despite the fact that only one woman in the interview group and very few outside were formally married in the 'traditional' sense, with *lobola* 'bride price' having been paid by the future husband to his father-in-law. There was also a marked absence of solidarity between female generations, and a distinct lack of reference to *abantu* 'community' as a possible source of support. This contrasts with the situation in the townships, where reference to *abantu* is ubiquitous, symbolizing a vibrant source of shared experience and political activism.

This absence of reference to *abantu* was in many ways surprising in a context in which NGOs are largely absent. The government on the other hand was seen as being the most likely source of help, something which a neoliberal reading might interpret as a dependency response. Community dynamics in the region are complex, however, and altogether different from the townships. The district is largely tribal trust land and Inkhata country, where interventions and decisions in the community are taken with reference to the local chief, or his representative, the *Induna*. These structures and political realities mean that political sensitivities and, above all, questions of confidentiality will limit the usefulness of conventionally favoured focus groups and other procedures which might otherwise have helped to triangulate on some of the findings. Detailed case studies over time would seem to be the most appropriate method of validation.

What conclusions maybe drawn from this small-scale study? And most importantly, despite its limited scope, what has the project achieved?

Conclusions

First, it is important to consider the wider applications of the storytelling technique. Since narrative forms are shared by all societies, this method has a potentially wider application in other health contexts when trying to envoice marginalized communities, including their perceptions and use of health services. Narratives can also be useful in training for a broader social ethic (Jones, 1997).

It is important too to consider how the marginalized knowledge elicited through interactive narrative might be fed back to policy makers and decision makers, and used beyond the formal policy context to challenge prevailing gender relations (Seidel 1996b). Might this perhaps lead over time to a men's group supporting the few men who may be in caring roles? And what of support for women who may not wish to be carers? Such developments, involving a no less important gender questioning process, would basically challenge assumptions about biologically based gender differences.

The role of 'outsiders', like more experienced advocacy groups not based in rural areas, raises sensitive issues such as, who speaks for whom? However, these are important challenges that are being addressed in the new South African political dispensation and the growing emphasis on the extension of women's rights, including women's reproductive and sexual health.[2]

What other forms of reflection linked to transformatory processes are suitable for use in rural areas? Other gender-sensitive participative techniques include practices developed by family planning groups to envoice and 'empower' women (e.g. KIT, 1995) and which use storyline techniques to invite women to reflect on their own lives, in some cases for the first time. Even in a safe environment, this can be a very emotional experience (Gordon, 1994).

Linking some of these best practices with forum theatre could offer a useful way forward, although inevitably this will be a slow process. Forum theatre as practised by Arturo Boal (1995), initially in Brazil, in the form of the Theatre of the Oppressed, is not a conventional, 'closed', authorial theatre. Based on Freirian techniques of 'learning from below' (Freire, 1983), it is scripted and rescripted in an interactive fashion. Spectators become *spect-actors* as they intervene and perform their own story, acting out solutions to their own local problems, including male violence. In Eritrea, for example, where such a technique has been used, these problems have focused on ownership and access to land, marriage and questions of inheritance. Such questions are no less central to women and the future of their children in the context of AIDS. HIV/AIDS is after all a development, gender and rights issue, not merely a biomedical phenomenon (Seidel, 1993).

A commitment to change presupposes some theory, such as social movements theory (Escobar, 1992). But theory, other than neoliberal thinking, has so far been disturbingly absent from the pragmatic, decontextualized, and medically led or medically designed interventions in the AIDS field. 'Empowerment', that ubiquitous elastic catchword (Baylies and Bujra, 1995), has been seen to consist simply of encouraging women to be more assertive in particular areas, by teaching them particular 'discursive technologies' (Seidel and Vidal, 1997). This ignores structural inequalities of power as part of a neoliberal market discourse of personal choice. More fundamentally, change needs to be seen as part of a larger political project that shifts the balance between women and men (Holland *et al.*, 1992; Kaijage, 1993) and challenges the androcentric bias (Fee, 1981; Doyal, 1996) and binary cultural constitution of gender.

This transformatory work is likely to involve new social actors. The use of forum theatre for development[3] has been hailed as a vehicle to encourage more participatory citizenship at a time when some NGOs and health professionals are seeking ways of challenging and organizing against some of the effects of globalization. This includes its impact on health and development (Lee and Zwi, 1996) as well as its gendered consequences (Table 4.1). In keeping with the commitments of the 1994 Reconstruction and Development Programme in South Africa, set out by the African National Congress (ANC), techniques such as interactive storytelling[4] combined with other participative frameworks seek to give primacy to the most dispossessed; that is, to rural women and the communities in which they live. In so doing, they aim to make new epistemological and interdisciplinary connections. This conceptualization is profoundly at odds with the 'short-termism' of much current research funding and of its concern with immediate quantifiable outcomes. It is also in tension with traditional top-down approaches to health and HIV education which have had little intersectoral relevance, and which have rarely engaged with the needs of non-literate rural communities. Moreover, where such approaches have sought to address women, it has been as educators, carers for men, or as vectors of infection (Strebel, 1995). Neoliberal approaches of this kind, with their emphasis on individualism and 'choice' make little sense, in development contexts. They are ahistorical, and seriously underestimate the centrality of social relations.

Table 4.1 Gender, equity, and improving care and access to care for the most marginalized rural women: how they have been carried through in this pilot study

- Focus on grassroots versus 'expert' knowledge
- Action research: elicit and use bottom-up knowledge and concerns to try to influence policy
- Improve the quality of care (epistemological and ethical dimensions of research)
- Problematize the meanings attached to 'community care' and 'care within the family' in gender terms (gender in development and equity concern)
- Use innovative methods and gendered parameters to elicit sensitive data not available through more conventional methods
- Network with related projects in the region, and with advocacy and human rights groups as social agents of change, and giving primacy to the building of civil society

Acknowledgements

This study was undertaken with a grant from the Nuffield Foundation. It was hosted by the Centre for Epidemiological Research in South Africa (CERSA) in Durban and Hlabisa. An associated workshop on gender and AIDS (Durban, July 1995), hosted by CERSA, Medical Research Council, Durban, was funded by a consultancy from the British Council. Gill Seidel would like to thank members of the HIV positive peer group and the entire AIDS team at Hlabisa, the regional NACOSA (National Convention of AIDS in South Africa), Slim Abdool-Karim, David Wilkinson (CERSA), Zama Nxumalo (CHESS), Alan Whiteside (University of Natal), the former Storyteller Group (Johannesburg) and Alan Jaffe at Amatikulu for their encouragement and support.

Notes

1 In a pilot study carried out elsewhere in the region, one woman became very excited by Zanile's story: 'How did you know this? This is my story!' Yet, curiously, one man, a former miner and hence migrant worker, claimed not to know any migrant workers when asked the question relating to identifying with Joseph's story. This highlights the problems of interpreting at any level, and underlines the enormous problems associated with large-scale and rapid surveys. Furthermore, how can this be done without 'mainstreaming' this knowledge since so often this has involved co-option of critical and gendered voices, including of women's associations (Hirschmann, 1991).

2 In South Africa the very active Association of Lawyers for Human Rights shares such concerns, as do women's rights and advocacy groups. These are accessible and they try to liaise, build connections, and move reflection and policy forward wherever abuses, including abuse of women and children, are brought to their attention.

3 The use of forum theatre would have training implications, and would benefit from south–south as well as north–south exchanges and experience of multilingual settings. This would involve training needs and research capacities as part of a longer process and vision of the use of theatre for development (TFD) (Plastow, 1997; Preston Whyte and Dalrymple, 1996).

4 Combining interactive storytelling with forum theatre has many implications. It could transform the parameters of more traditional fieldwork. It is also very helpful even when baseline data is lacking, or inadequate, and especially where there is no gender disaggregation. Eliciting a 'thicker context' using more conventional anthropological techniques and other methods to elicit reliable ethnographic data about social relations and gender calls for adequate training, time and the building of trust. An additional difficulty is that, in development contexts, a number of qualified researchers

(social scientists and health professionals) may have limited fluency in regional languages, and especially in local language varieties. And it is not unusual, given the demanding nature of rural fieldwork and its other deprivations, for it to be subcontracted to inexperienced fieldworkers, and directed from a distance, since rural work is perceived by urban professionals as being of low status. This may lead to gaps and inaccuracies which may go unchallenged, and which may be used as a basis for policy recommendations.

References

ARMSTRONG, S. (1994) 'Rape – an invisible part of apartheid's legacy', in Sweetman, C. (ed.) *Population and Reproductive Rights*. London: Zed Books.

BAKHTIN, M. (1981) *The Dialogic Imagination*. Austin, TX: University of Texas Press.

BAYLIES, C. and BUJRA, J. (1995) 'Discourses of power and empowerment in the fight against HIV/AIDS in Africa', in Aggleton, P., Davies, P. and Hart, G. (eds) *AIDS: Safety, Sexuality and Risk*. London: Taylor & Francis.

BOAL, A. (1995) *The Rainbow of Desire*. London: Routledge.

COLEMAN, R. (1996) 'The role of traditional medical practitioners in the prevention and management of HIV disease', *AIDS Analysis Africa*, **6**, pp. 5–7.

DOYAL, L. (1996) 'The politics of women's health', *International Journal of Health Services*, **26**, 1, pp. 47–65.

ESCOBAR, A. (1992) 'Culture, practice and politics: anthropology and the study of social movements', *Critique of Anthropology*, **12**, 4, pp. 395–432.

FEE, E. (1981) 'Is feminism a threat to scientific objectivity?', *International Journal of Women's Studies*, **4**, pp. 213–33.

FRANK, A.W. (1995) *The Wounded Storyteller: Body, Illness and Ethics*. Chicago, IL: Chicago University Press.

FREIRE, P. (1983) *Education for Critical Consciousness*. New York: Seabury Press and Continuum Press.

GORDON, G. (1994) 'Drawing a sexual lifeline', *Health Action*, Sept/Nov, pp. 6–7.

HEISE, L. and ELIAS, C. (1995) 'Transforming AIDS prevention to meet women's needs: a focus on developing countries', *Social Science and Medicine*, **40**, pp. 931–43.

HIRSCHMANN, D. (1991) 'Women and political participation in Africa: broadening the scope of research', *World Development*, **19**, 12, pp. 1679–94.

HOLLAND, J. *et al.* (1992) 'Pressure, resistance, empowerment: young women and the negotiation of safer sex', in Aggleton, P., Davies, P. and Hart, G. (eds) *AIDS: Rights, Risk and Reason*. London: Falmer Press.

HYDEN, L.-C. (1997) 'Illness and narrative', *Sociology of Health and Illness*, **19**, 1, pp. 48–69.

HYMES, D. (1996) *Ethnography, Linguistics, Narrative Inequality – Towards an Understanding of Voice*. London: Taylor & Francis.

JONES, A.H. (1997) 'Literature and medicine: narrative ethics', *Lancet*, **349**, p. 1243.

KAIJAGE, T. (1993) 'People striving to control the spread of AIDS', in Berer, M. and Ray, S. (eds) *Women and HIV/AIDS: An International Resource Book*. London: Pandora.

KIT (Royal Tropical Institute) (1995) *Facing the Challenges of STDs, HIV/ AIDS: A Gender-Based Response*. Amsterdam: KIT, WHO and SAFAIDS.

LEE, K. and ZWI, A.B. (1996) 'A global political economy approach to AIDS: ideology, interests and implications', *New Political Economy*, **1**, 3, pp. 355–73.

MOORE, H.L. (1994) *A Passion for Difference*. Cambridge: Polity Press.

PLASTOW, J. (1997) *Follow-up to the Theatre-and-Development Seminar, The Barbican, London, 23 March 1997*. Report of the Workshop Theatre, University of Leeds.

PRESTON-WHYTE, E. and DALRYMPLE, L. (1996) 'Participation and action: reflections on community-based AIDS interventions in South Africa', in de Koning, K. and Martin, M. (eds) *Participatory Research in Health*. London: Zed Books.

RAYNAUT, C. (1996) 'Quelles questions pour la discipline? Quelle collaboration avec la médecine, in Benoist, J. and Desclaux, A. (eds) *Anthropologie et SIDA*. Paris: Editions Karthala.

ROSS, S.M., NXUMALO, Z. and PHILPOTT, R.H. (1994) *Situation Analysis of a Home-based Care Scheme for HIV/AIDS*. Durban: University of Natal Community Health, Education and Support Service (CHESS).

ROTHERBERG, K.H. and PASKEY, S.J. (1995) 'The risk of domestic violence and women with HIV infection: implications for partner notification, public policy and law', *American Journal of Public Health*, **85**, 11, pp. 1569–76.

SEIDEL, G. (1993) 'The competing discourses of HIV/AIDS in sub-Saharan Africa', *Social Science and Medicine*, **36**, 3, pp. 175–94.

SEIDEL, G. (1995) Stories in many languages – some ways forward for STD and AIDS education in the new South Africa. *Sociétés d'Afrique et SIDA*, **6**, Oct.

SEIDEL, G. (1996a) 'Confidentiality and HIV status in KwaZulu-Natal: implications, resistances, challenges', *Health Policy and Planning*, **11**, 4, pp. 418–27.

SEIDEL, G. (1996b) 'Seeking to optimise care for HIV positive women and extending the gendered rights' discourse – conceptualising the dilemmas, with illustrations from fieldwork in rural KwaZulu-Natal'. Paper presented to the International Symposium on Social Sciences and AIDS in Africa, Senegal, 4–8 November, 1996.

SEIDEL, G. and NTULI, N. (1996) 'HIV confidentiality, gender and support in KwaZulu-Natal', *Lancet*, **347**, p. 469.

SEIDEL, G. and VIDAL, L. (1997) 'The implications of "medical", "gender in development" and "culturalist" discourses for HIV/AIDS policy in Africa', in Shore, C. and Wright, S. (eds) *Anthropology of Policy*. London: Routledge.

SOLDAN, K., ABDOOL-KARIM, Q. and ABDOOL-KARIM, S. (1994) *Home-based Care for HIV/AIDS: Evaluation of the KwaZulu Pilot Programme*. Durban: Medical Research Council.

STREBEL, A. (1995) *The Discourses of Women and AIDS in South Africa*. PhD thesis, Department of Psychology, University of the Western Cape.

TEMMERMAN, M. *et al.* (1995) 'The right not to know HIV test results', *Lancet*, **345**, pp. 969–70.

WOOD, K., MAFORAH, F. and JEWKES, R. (1996) *Sex, Violence and Constructions of Love among Xhosa Adolescents: Putting Violence on the Sexuality Education Agenda*, Tygerberg, South Africa: CERSA Women's Health, Medical Research Council.

Chapter 5

Narratives of Care, Love and Commitment: AIDS/HIV and Non-Heterosexual Family Formations

Brian Heaphy, Jeffrey Weeks and Catherine Donovan

Situated historically in a period of discourse on lesbian and gay kinship, AIDS has served as an impetus to establish and expand gay families. In certain cases, blood relations joined with gay friends and relatives to assist the chronically ill or dying. Sometimes a family of friends was transformed into a group of caregivers with ties to one another as well as the persons with AIDS. Community organizations have begun to offer counselling to persons with AIDS 'and their loved ones', while progressive hospitals and hospices modified residence and visitation policies to embrace 'family as the client defines family'. Implicit in a phrase like 'loved ones' is an open-ended notion of kinship that respects the principles of choice and self-determination in defining kin, with love spanning the ideologically contrasting domains of biological family and the families we create (Weston, 1991).

While the above quotation refers to the relationship between AIDS/HIV and lesbian and gay family life in San Francisco in the late 1980s, it touches on some of the key themes addressed in this chapter on AIDS/HIV and non-heterosexual family forms in Britain today. These include the complex and fluid nature of terms such as 'family' and 'friends' when they are employed to tell stories of non-heterosexual relationships, the notion that kinship can somehow be about choice and self-determination, and the extent to which we must expand our definitions of family if we are to fully understand the 'familial' aspects of AIDS/HIV.

In the literature, AIDS has been located as a potential catalyst in expanding definitions of family to reflect the reality of contemporary life (e.g. Levine, 1991). It has also been argued that responses to the epidemic have made non-heterosexual caring relationships more visible (e.g. Adam, 1992), and have allowed gay 'extended families' to demonstrate their strength and durability (e.g. Bronski, 1988). It has further been suggested that such relationships may be stronger and more durable than traditional family forms as they are built on support and respect, and are chosen (Bronski, 1988; Plummer, 1995). There has, however, been very little systematic research on what we term 'families of choice' which can be employed to evaluate or make sense of such claims (for a review of the literature see Weeks, Donovan and Heaphy, 1996).

In this chapter we draw from our own research on non-heterosexual family formations to explore this crucial aspect of local responses to AIDS/ HIV that has been widely mentioned in the literature, but has rarely been worked out in any detail.[1] Focusing on in-depth interviews with gay men, lesbians and bisexuals across Britain, we argue that consideration of the familial aspects of AIDS/HIV must include 'new' or emerging stories of non-heterosexual 'families of choice' that emphasize the themes of mutual care, love and commitment.

Non-Heterosexual Family Stories

Throughout our research on non-heterosexual relationships, our concern has been with 'new' narratives and ways of conceiving family and intimate life (see Heaphy, Donovan and Weeks, 1998). Stories, Plummer suggests, significantly shape the ways in which we conceive of social life:

> Society itself may be seen as a textured but seamless web of stories emerging everywhere through interaction ... the metaphor of the story ... has become recognised as one of the central roots we have into the continuing quest for understanding human meaning. (Plummer 1995: 5)

New stories about family and intimate life emerge when there is a new audience ready to hear them, and when newly vocal groups can have their experiences validated by them. They, in turn, are enabled to retell the stories in ever burgeoning ways, and this in turn gives rise to new demands for recognition and validation as the new narratives circulate.

While one major story of our time has been that of the traditional heterosexual nuclear family, stories are now beginning to emerge regarding non-heterosexual family forms (Plummer, 1995). Lesbian and gay communities may constitute a relatively small part of the contemporary ecology of social life, but in recent years they have been the focus of strong social and political controversy, particularly with regard to what can be broadly termed 'family' issues. In Britain in the late 1980s the relationship between 'gay' and 'family' became the focus of popular discourse because of concern with the legitimacy of 'pretended families' (Weeks, 1991). Debates over the age of consent continue to raise questions of equal rights, as do ever increasing debates about same-sex marriage and partnership rights. Issues to do with parenting, including lesbian and gay adoption, surrogacy and self-insemination, continue to be high profile, and appear to be the cause of much political and media anxiety. Such concerns might be related to broader concerns and anxieties that have focused on the decline of the 'traditional' family. Yet, our own research suggests that while traditional forms may be changing, the language of family is very much alive, not least among the groups of people, lesbians and gay men particularly, who have been seen in the past as the very antithesis of traditional family life.

It is not, however, only the *language* of family that is alive and thriving among some lesbians and gay men. Rather, we would argue, the use of this language is suggestive of a strong perceived need for the sort of values and comforts that have been associated with the traditional ideal of family. For many lesbians and gay men, including many of our research subjects, the need and desire for such values and comforts have been accentuated in the age of AIDS/HIV. This is particularly evident with regard to issues of care for the sick and the dying. AIDS/HIV has also highlighted questions of values in a broader sense, particularly in terms of formal and informal recognition of relationships, and the extension of familial rights to those who are chosen as family.

Families of Choice

It has been widely noted that 'coming out' as lesbian or gay to family of origin can result in a distancing from parents and siblings who are disillusioned and disappointed, and at the most extreme it can result in rejection by family of origin (e.g. Muller, 1987; Davies, 1992; Marcus 1992). Conversely, it has been suggested that *not* coming out can also distance non-heterosexuals from kin (Driggs and Finn, 1991; Cramer and Roach, 1988). From such accounts it could be argued that the often presumed mutual exclusivity of 'gay' and 'family' means that lesbians and gay men have no choice but to create 'surrogate' or 'pretend' families in an attempt to replace estranged kin. A similar argument has been extended to the family networks of people living with AIDS/HIV (PWA/HIV), where it is argued that PWA/HIV, and particularly gay men with AIDS/HIV, may *have* to acquire new family for emotional and economic support due to the fact that AIDS/HIV can cause intrafamilial rifts (Levine, 1991). However, we want to suggest here that there is another way of looking at the topic: for many people these 'new' families should be seen in terms of *choice* and *agency* rather than desperate need. While it is the case that careworkers, volunteers and 'professionals' may fulfil some of the functions of family for PWA/HIV, and may be termed 'surrogate' families, they must be distinguished from 'intentional' (Cruikshank 1992) or 'chosen' (Weston, 1991) forms.

In this sense it is becoming increasingly acknowledged that for many people today, both heterosexual and non-heterosexual, 'family' does not apply only to relationships that are linked to biology and blood or the unit created by legally sanctioned marriage (Weston, 1991; Plummer, 1995; Weeks, Donovan and Heaphy, 1996). In the family stories being told at the end of the twentieth century there is a sense that, for some people, family is something you create for yourself, something that involves interactions, commitments and responsibilities that are negotiated in a world where few things are given or certain. From our research on non-heterosexual 'family-type' relationships it would appear that this is certainly the case for many lesbians and gay men. As one respondent put it:

> So one of the things I learned when I came out as a lesbian was that I have the right to create my own family – a new family that, like a 'family of choice' rather than a family that I'd just been born into. And so I see those few friends as being my new family. And so they're absolutely and fundamentally important to me in terms of supporting me and giving me all the things that I want from people in order to survive. (Respondent F03; all female interviews are denoted by F, all male interviews by M)

Among many self-identified lesbians and gay men the term 'family' is frequently used to denote something broader than family of origin: an affinity circle which has cultural and symbolic meaning for the subjects that participate or feel a sense of belonging through it. In our research the most commonly used terms for these elective families were 'chosen' or 'created'. Such terms form part of a narrative of invention which is very powerful among our respondents. Such a notion was frequently expressed with regard to both 'self identity' and 'relationships':

> Speaking for my generation, you know – my age – discovering that I was homosexual meant having to invent myself because there was nothing there that . . . there weren't any role models there. It may well be different for gay men coming out now, I don't know. . . . But there's still that element of self-invention and finding . . . defining things how you want them to be. (M17)

> I think it's actually a better lifestyle. . . . Because you have to think about it all the time. So nothing you do is ever just following the set pattern that someone . . . you know, it's not set down . . . I mean I know it's all very restrained by the sort of oppressions out there but within a group of lesbians and gay men, you get to choose the way you want to behave and you're not restrained by stupid bloody conventions. (M11)

Accounts such as the above are evident in many coming-out stories (e.g. Hall Carpenter Archives, 1989a; 1989b; Porter and Weeks, 1990), and the extent to which self-invention is central to lesbian and gay experience has been widely noted in the literature on lesbian and gay identity (Weston, 1991; Plummer, 1992; 1995; Blasius, 1994; Weeks, 1995). So it is not surprising that in interviews concerning the intimate lives of non-heterosexuals these themes should be extended to the necessity or possibility of creating and choosing family-type relationships. However, some recent work has argued that engaging in 'everyday experiments', with regard to creating and choosing relationships, is now a common experience for both heterosexuals and non-heterosexuals (Giddens, 1992; Bech, 1996).

From the accounts of non-heterosexuals, the notion of choice with regard to family life emerges most strongly in stories of friends and partners *being* family or being *like* family. Among our respondents, the vast majority of those who were in couple relationships considered their partners to be part of their family networks. Also, while many of those interviewed talked about friendships as being very similar to family relationships, others emphasized the extent to which friends *were* family (Nardi, 1992a). In both types of account, friendship circles (which were often inclusive of partners) were often presented as idealized family, offering such things as 'companionship, love, respect' (M04), together with practical and material support. As the following respondents put it:

> [Closest friendships] are important to me because they've been with me a long time and through a lot of stuff . . . and we've been quite a support to each other, helping each other out, sorting out childcare. If I'm ill or if I need help, they'll give it. . . . I suppose in a way they're my family. (F40)

> It's a kind of stability. A kind of solid rock. I suppose. . . . You can just be with them and be yourself, and it's great because they love you just the way you are. . . . And I think the fact that, that you can rely on them in times of need, as well. And that's mutual. That if you had a phone call that someone was upset or something bad had happened or someone needed help financially, whatever . . . no question, you know. (M32)

Relationships with friends and partners are often described as being more reliable that those with biological or legal kin. One female respondent implied this when she noted that her friends were 'supportive, and understand in a way that your family should and often doesn't' (F43). Friends and partners were widely described as providing 'in general' what family is thought to, or 'should' provide:

> I suppose in a romantic sense or in a personal sense anyway, I get what families do for each other, I think, from my relationship with my boyfriend and from my friends. (M05)

> They're my lifeline. Yes. And particularly, as I said earlier, my family don't offer that. I couldn't survive without my friends. (F44)

Accounts such as these are in line with the limited literature on non-heterosexual friendship relationships; this suggests they offer a special bonding that is central in the maintenance of self and identity among the members of marginalized groups (Rubin, 1985); a network or group which provides for 'being oneself' in a cultural context that may not approve of that self (Nardi, 1992a); confirmation of people's self-identity, in providing practical and emotional support (Nardi, 1992b; Nardi and Sherrod, 1994); belonging and nurturance (Raphael and Robinson, 1984); and emotional support, sustenance and commitment (Becker, 1992: 164). Among our respondents, terms such as 'love' and 'trust' were widely employed to sum up the central qualities of friendships and friendship families:

> Love and trust are the two things that are most important about what I get from [friends], that I know that I trust them, they trust me, I love them, they love me and that sense of really, it's not that love you get with your family [of origin], it's that I know they like me as well. So they've chose it. You know, in a way that you can't possibly choose it with your family [of origin]. (M11)

Some writers have suggested that kin is a common metaphor for describing closeness between friends due to the lack of a readily available language to describe central associations that are not related to blood or legal connections (Rubin, 1985). It is not, however, that 'everybody counts' (Levine 1991). Rather, the emphasis is placed on *particular* relationships, where commitments have been negotiated and worked out over time, and this is similar to shifts noted in wider heterosexual kin relationships (Finch and Mason, 1993). This brings up an important point with regard to definitions of family. While certain friends may be identified as being family, and while members of couple relationships may overwhelmingly identify partners as part of their family networks, accepting members of family of origin can also be included in definitions of a family of choice. In this sense, family of origin and family of choice are not necessarily mutually exclusive, as inclusion in the family of choice tends to depend on the quality of the relationship, irrespective of the biological tie (Weston, 1991). This is indicated in the following extract from one respondent's account of who it is that counts as family:

> My friends – to some extent my sister and my father, but I think because I like them. If I didn't like them . . . I wouldn't be at all sure. But my friends, my lovers, yes. (F34)

Some recent studies (e.g. Roberts and McGlone, 1997) suggest that most people still make a basic distinction between friends and kin in terms of the key areas of obligation and commitment. However, for many non-heterosexuals such circles provide more than the term 'friendship' usually denotes, even if it is the case that commitment is not measured in terms of obligation. Rather, the emphasis is placed on a mutual responsibility for working out the relationship. Indeed, the term obligation has negative implications for many. As one respondent put it:

> I've tried to avoid the sense of [familial] obligation with my friendships – you know – that it's kind of like that they're there because they want to be there. If they like me, well . . . don't have any obligations . . . I've changed what didn't work for me in my natural family when I was growing up, I . . . I've replaced it with something that does work, within my friendships. I think that's the difference. I've chosen quite carefully. (M33)

We would stress here that there are important limits on choice. Choices are contingent on many factors, constrained by the socioeconomic, cultural and historical contexts in which we live (Weston, 1991). The most important factor, however, may not be the limits, real as they are, but the ethos that stories of non-heterosexual friendship reveal: that a sense of self-worth and cultural confidence is realized in and through families of choice. Such rewards may make the creation and maintaining of such commitments a worthwhile endeavour, even if the responsibility this entails is often perceived to involve more labour than traditional relationships based on obligation and set expectations. As one respondent put it when talking of the value of friendship:

> They're more . . . in some ways perhaps they're more important than family, because I mean, I don't like to say it but I think the fact is, I take my family for granted, whereas my friendships are, to a degree, chosen and therefore created. And I feel a greater responsibility to nourish them and try to maintain them. (M21)

Chosen Relationships and AIDS/HIV

In the accounts gathered for our research, narratives of chosen relationships and families of choice often overlap with narratives of the impact of AIDS/HIV. This is particularly the case with regard to the stories of gay men. In such accounts AIDS/HIV is presented in various ways as a moment of crisis, with implications at individual, community and familial levels. In this sense AIDS/HIV appears to be experienced, in different ways, as a 'fateful moment' (Heaphy, 1996). Giddens describes such moments in the following way:

> Fateful moments are times when events come together in such a way that an individual stands, as it were, at a crossroads in his

> existence. . . . There are, of course, fateful moments in the history of
> collectives as well as in the lives of individuals. They are phases at
> which things are wrenched out of joint, where a given state of affairs
> is suddenly altered by a few key events. (Giddens, 1991: 113)

Such moments mark times of change for those affected, be they individuals
or groups, and as such often necessitate 'reskilling' (or relearning) and 're-
evaluation' in an endeavour to make sense of the 'new' situation. For most
of the gay male respondents we interviewed, AIDS/HIV appears to have
necessitated a 'reskilling' in the form of efforts to become familiar with both
safer sex information and AIDS/HIV knowledge in a broader sense. For many
of those who were sexually active before the advent of AIDS/HIV, such
reskilling has in turn led to a 'rethinking' of their sexual lives, particularly with
regard to the practising of safer sex.

It is noteworthy that while the vast majority of our gay male respondents
stated they practised what they understood to be safer sex, a small number of
those who described themselves as being in committed couple relationships
did not. Following from work such as that of Prieur (1990), Davies *et al.* (1993)
and Henriksson (1995), we would suggest that in such contexts the temptation
to characterize 'unsafe' sex as an irrational act is of limited value. Rather, it
may be more productive to attempt to understand such acts in the terms of
couple narratives of love, commitment and trust. As Henriksson (1995) notes,
in the context of unprotected anal sex, the giving and receiving of semen can
have symbolic meaning for some gay men, and can signify a symbolic border
between 'casual' and 'real' relations. In the stories told in our research, unprotected anal sex was reserved for the central relationship, and was often presented as both an indicator and expression of trust. For some of those in
non-monogamous relationships, like the respondent below, the decision to
practice 'unsafe' sex had come about as a result of explicit negotiations with
the central partner, and was presented as a marker of the 'specialness' of the
primary relationship:

> Ultimately I think what we were both talking about was a sense
> of trust between us and the fact that here was something special
> between us that we wouldn't do with other people . . . we both of us
> have a fair amount of sex with other men, anyway, somehow it makes
> the sex between us more special as well. (M25)

If the focus on narratives of love and commitment can help us to make sense
of this, in a broad sense these narratives flow into wider notions of care and
support in the context of AIDS/HIV. At one level such themes are evident in
accounts of both gay men's and lesbians' caring responses to the crisis, which
are framed in terms of commitments that flow from a sense of belonging to
some 'community':

This sounds really crass but it was just simply I wanted to go and do something about something that was happening to a community that I belong to. And yes I wanted to be educated. I wanted more information but I also wanted to do something positive which ... whatever I could do. That's it in a nutshell, really, I think for me. (M06)

I think it's a feeling of being part of a community and ... I ... I see ... you know I just see us as part of a group who are in a minority, and we need to support each other very, very much and I would like to support anyone who was HIV or with AIDS. (F05)

Even for those gay men and lesbians who have not experienced the impact of the virus and syndrome at the level of friendship or family, the impact at the level of community appears to have facilitated an engagement with issues to do with caring commitments at a very personal level. As the extract below indicates, the impact at community and individual levels can be closely linked in this regard:

I think it ... has affected the lesbian and gay community ... and I think it has a ... it does have that kind of impact. That sort of ... it does make you think about all those issues about caring. About what would happen if you became chronically ill. All that stuff about death ... all the taboo subjects. (F27)

Many of the accounts of our respondents contain evidence of the extent to which the collective fateful moment of AIDS/HIV has necessitated both a collective and individual engagement with the 'taboo' subjects identified by the respondent above. AIDS/HIV has brought up questions of care for others, but as the following extract demonstrates, it also highlights issues of care for the self:

We both have friends who have been very ill and friends who have died – of AIDS. And we ... we've actually discussed it with them, that we would be quite happy for them to come and stay with us and that extended to what would happen if it was one of us. ... We'd probably be able to have a nurse or somebody to come in during the day – but we'd be at home and we'd care for each other. (M04)

Though many of those within couple relationships tend to negotiate the possibilities and practicalities of care for each other with partners, wider friendship circles or families of choice still figure highly in accounts of potential providers of care. In these accounts the emphasis is placed on the reciprocal nature of such commitments. It is also worth noting that within some circles particular individuals may sometimes be identified, or identify themselves, as 'the carer'. Such individuals may not only provide informal care for friends, but also to members of the broader 'gay community'. Though relatively few of these individuals were identified in our research, this extract from one interview describes such a friend:

> He has taken younger boys under his wing. . . . And he's had three AIDS sufferers whom he's taken into his home and looked after, and he's got one at the moment. I mean, he's not there all the time but you know, he more or less says, 'Feel free to stay here whenever you want, whenever you need to. Whenever you need peace and quiet or whatever.' And so he does that. So, if I were chronically ill and Lindon weren't able to care for me or whatever, Wayne – even though he is so much older, and, you know, luckily he's fit for his age . . . I'm sure he would. (M36)

In the end, accounts of the impact of AIDS/HIV at the level of friendship or family are consistently framed in terms of fateful moments, where caring responses flow 'naturally' from the nature of the relationship:

> Certainly with individual friends who have been sick and dying, you know, I suppose when we've been involved [in caring] . . . it seems to be when somebody gets sick or when somebody dies – through necessity or just through circumstances rather than making an effort to get involved on a general level, or a general basis. (M37)

The Value of Relationships

Friendships flourish, it has been argued, when overarching identities are fragmented in periods of rapid social change, or at crucial moments in individual lives (Weeks, 1995). Indeed, accounts of the impact of AIDS/HIV on friendship or family networks provide evidence of the extent to which the epidemic has led many individuals to re-evaluate the importance of these particular relationships:

> I think it makes you appreciate your friends more. You know, when you start losing your friends you start looking at the friends you've got left, and you really value what they have to offer you. (F14)

> I am more aware of people, of feelings. I am more aware of the importance of friendship – of relationships. I am more aware of the need for trust, and being dependable. . . . When people around us

have died – you know, the people that we have known – the love has been there to start with. And as I said before, you know – when you've got that relationship with somebody there's ... you know – there's something inside that tells you there is more love needed or less love needed. You need to be more involved or less involved. You need to be more supportive or less supportive. I think that's always been there and I think that I think AIDS/HIV has specifically made it more important as far as friends are concerned. (M04)

As the extracts above indicate, making sense of the impact of AIDS/HIV can often involve a reassessment of the value of particular friendship or family relationships. It is not, however, that AIDS/HIV has introduced the possibilities of love, support and care into such relationships. Rather, it appears to have highlighted the existence and necessity of these for many people. In this sense the experience of AIDS/HIV can work to accentuate and facilitate a recognition of the value of relationships at this level. AIDS/HIV may highlight issues of care and the value of chosen relationships, but we would also stress that for many non-heterosexual families and friendship networks, these issues can arise in the context of other crises and fateful moments. For members of such groups, broader concerns with care, e.g. those that arise with regard to ageing, can necessitate a collective working out of various possibilities and the making explicit of commitments to each other:

[We've] begun to think about, 'Well, how could we organize things in such a way that we can look after ourselves?' ... We do talk about the future and how we would look after each other. ... In all of it, there's something sort of 'collective' about everybody pooling their resources in some way in order to sustain us all ... we've got to ... it's got to be sensible to do some kind of 'pooling' idea. (M11)

If the value of chosen relationships can be accentuated at times of crisis, some of our respondents' accounts of the impact of AIDS/HIV highlight the extent to which such relationships might also be *devalued* at a broader level. Stories of the importance of friends and families of choice being denied recognition at times of illness and death were not uncommon among those interviewed. The following quotation from a respondent recounting the impact of the death of a friend provides one such account:

I think it's had a fairly major impact, really. But not in an immediately obvious way. Because it was around for a long time and I knew his HIV status for about ten years – and he's kind of never actually had any major illnesses for about eight of those years that I've known him ... his family weren't really at ease with the fact that he was HIV

Brian Heaphy, Jeffrey Weeks and Catherine Donovan

positive. And when he died the biggest impact was that they didn't
tell anybody that he died – and they had the funeral very quickly and
didn't invite any of his . . . his friends. You know, that was like
their . . . the impact it had on me was kind of being more determined
to be myself and. . . . Not to have – not to allow my family to do that.
(M33)

For many the lack of both formal and informal recognition of same-sex
partnerships and non-traditional family relationships has been made more
explicit in the context of AIDS/HIV. For some of our interviewees these issues
arose most dramatically at times of death. At such times the 'automatic' rights
of families of origin, whatever their relationships to the deceased, was often
most emphasized. Recognition of the importance of other relationships, and
the reality of non-heterosexual lives, often depends on the goodwill of the
family of origin. In the following quotation a lesbian respondent refers to
the death of a gay male friend:

You should have a right to have a say in each other's health care.
If your partner was hospitalized, you should have the same right as
any other partner would have – and that goes for whether you're
straight or gay, you know. Not a lot of straights get married these
days and there should be equal rights for everyone. We should
all have a say in what happens – say with funeral things. I mean
Sam's funeral was *horrific*. His parents completely took over; his
boyfriend was hardly mentioned or . . . or spoken to, and it was a
very Christian burial. It was hideous. Absolutely nothing to do with
his life – the preacher didn't know him and just stood reading from
a piece of paper. And because his parents preferred his female
friends, they had a bigger say in what happened than his partner did.
(F14)

For some, experiences such as these have brought home the importance
of being more explicit about the importance of chosen relationships. This
was clear when respondents talked of the importance of employing the legal
possibilities that were available, such as wills and so on, as a strategy in
acknowledging the reality of their own lives and relationships. Others, such as
the respondent below, adopt a less formal approach. Asked 'What about
funeral arrangements – have you ever made any provision for those?' he
replied:

Well, I've actually written stuff down – and actually some friends
have got it – but it's not like – it changes all the time, in fact. I
mean, I want . . . my parents are aware that I want a non-religious
ceremony. . . . I think my friends would want something completely
different. I went to this guy – the other guy who had AIDS and died

recently – his funeral was like the best . . . the best funeral I've ever been to. I know it's a contradiction in terms, but it was. It really made you think about who he was and what he meant to different people in his life – and it was a brilliant experience. And I'd like something like that . . . he'd got his friends . . . to come up and talk about what he meant to them, and what kind of things they'd done. . . . And you got a really clear picture about who he was and what his life was about. (M33)

For many respondents, AIDS/HIV has provided a lens through which 'inequality', 'discrimination', and the cultural privileging of heterosexuality were often viewed. In this sense, questions of recognition in terms of AIDS/HIV, and the related contexts of caring and death, were seen to be bound up with broader questions of rights and citizenship. With regard to recognition of couple relationships, while 'marriage' is certainly not to all tastes, politically and otherwise, there was broad agreement about having the same 'rights' and 'recognitions' as afforded to heterosexuals. As one respondent put it:

I think it's important . . . that we have equal legal rights with everyone else. Not necessarily marriage, but recognition that, you know, if Frankie was ill – terminally ill or something – that I would be recognized as her next of kin. (F40)

Among respondents who were involved in parenting, there was also an acute awareness of the potential problems that can arise at times of illness and death, where the 'rights' of same-sex partners to adopt or care for a child are easily contested. The extent to which there were few possibilities available with regard to the legal recognition of same-sex co-parenting relationships was emphasized by many. As one parent put it:

I mean the whole issue, just around legal custody as well – because the fact is, Frankie hasn't got any legal status with Lisa at the moment, so if anything happened to me, Frankie would have no rights . . . that makes me really angry, as well, that Frankie could spend years and years working around helping to raise, bring her up, and then if anything happens to me, you know, she's got no rights. (F40)

While questions of 'relational' rights and recognitions do not *only* arise in terms of AIDS/HIV, the epidemic has made these more urgent for many non-heterosexuals. As noted earlier, while AIDS/HIV has allowed many gay men and lesbians to re-evaluate and reassert their commitments to a broad set of chosen relationships, it has also clarified the extent to which these commitments might be denied in the wider culture.

Conclusions

In this chapter we have suggested that consideration of the familial aspects of AIDS/HIV must include 'new' or emerging stories of non-heterosexual 'families of choice' that emphasize the themes of mutual care, love and commitment. To do so is to engage with the potentially complex and fluid nature of terms such as 'family' and 'friends', and to acknowledge that kinship is not only about blood and legal ties, but can also be about choice and self-determination. In expanding our definitions of family, we can more fully understand the implications that AIDS/HIV has for family life, and make sense of local caring responses to the virus and syndrome.

In terms of the impact of AIDS/HIV, it is not that this 'fateful moment' has introduced concepts of love, care and commitment into non-heterosexual relationships, but rather it has accentuated the value of a range of chosen relationships for many. However, issues related to care and death in the context of AIDS/HIV can also highlight the extent to which such relationships are devalued at the broader level of formal and informal recognition. In the realm of policy relating to family and care, we would argue that dominant notions of 'who counts' do not match with the realities of emotional life for many people today.

The narratives of chosen relationships and AIDS/HIV highlighted here demonstrate that legislation and policies based on assumptions of the primacy of 'traditional' relations are in tension with such realities. Key dilemmas arise concerning the possibility of developing legislation and policy around more flexible definitions of what it is that constitutes family and family life. While the need for such flexibility has been acknowledged in some local AIDS/HIV contexts, wider changes in policy and social policy are required if the implications of families of choice are to be more fully recognized.

Note

1 This paper is based on research conducted for a project funded by the Economic and Social Research Council, entitled 'Families of Choice: The Structure and Meanings of Non-Heterosexual Relationships' (Ref. L315253030). The director of the project was Jeffrey Weeks; Catherine Donovan and Brian Heaphy were research fellows. The core of the research involved in-depth interviews with 48 men and 48 women who broadly identified as non-heterosexual (gay, lesbian, queer, bisexual, etc.).

References

Adam, B.D. (1992) 'Sex and caring among men', in Plummer, K. (ed.) *Modern Homosexualities: Fragments of Lesbian and Gay Experience*. London: Routledge.

BECH, H. (1996) *When Men Meet: Homosexuality and Modernity.* Cambridge: Polity Press.

BECKER, C.S. (1992) *Living and Relating: An Introduction to Phenomenology.* London: Sage.

BLASIUS, M. (1994) *Gay and Lesbian Politics: Sexuality and the Emergence of a New Ethic.* Philadelphia, PA: Temple University Press.

BRONSKI, M. (1988) 'Death and the erotic imagination', in Preston, J. (ed.) *Personal Dispatches: Writers Confront AIDS.* New York: St Martin's Press.

CRAMER, D.W. and ROACH, A.J. (1988) 'Coming out to mom and dad: a story of gay males and their relationships with parents', *Journal of Homosexuality*, **15**, pp. 79–92.

CRUIKSHANK, M. (1992) *The Lesbian and Gay Liberation Movement.* New York: Routledge.

DAVIES, P. (1992) 'The role of disclosure in coming out among gay men', in Plummer, K. (ed.) *Modern Homosexualities: Fragments of Lesbian and Gay Experience.* London: Routledge.

DAVIES, P.M., HICKSON, F.C., WEATHERBURN, P. and HUNT, A.J. (1993) *Sex, Gay Men and AIDS.* London: Falmer Press.

DRIGGS, J.H. and FINN, S.E. (1991) *Intimacy Between Men: How to Find and Keep Gay Love Relationships.* London: Plume.

FINCH, J. and MASON, J. (1993) *Negotiating Family Responsibilities.* London: Routledge.

GIDDENS, A. (1991) *Modernity and Self-Identity: Self and Society in the Late Modern Age.* Cambridge: Polity Press.

GIDDENS, A. (1992) *The Transformation of Intimacy: Sexuality, Love and Eroticism in Modern Societies.* Cambridge: Polity Press.

HALL CARPENTER ARCHIVES (1989a) *Inventing Ourselves: Lesbian Life Stories.* London: Routledge.

HALL CARPENTER ARCHIVES (1989b) *Walking After Midnight: Gay Men's Lifestories.* London: Routledge.

HEAPHY, B. (1996) 'Medicalisation and identity formation: identity and strategy in the context of AIDS and HIV', in Weeks, J. and Holland, J. (eds) *Sexual Cultures: Communities, Values and Intimacy.* London: Macmillan.

HEAPHY, B., DONOVAN, C. and WEEKS, J. (1998) '"That's like my life": researching stories of non-heterosexual relationships', *Sexualities*, **4**,(1), pp. 453–70.

HENRIKSSON, B. (1995) *Risk Factor Love: Homosexuality, Sexual Interaction and HIV Prevention.* PhD thesis, Department of Social Work, Gothenburg University, Sweden.

LEVINE, C. (1991) 'AIDS and changing concepts of family', in Nelkin, D., Willis, D.P. and Parris, S.V. (eds) *A Disease of Society: Cultural and Institutional Responses to AIDS.* New York: Cambridge University Press.

Brian Heaphy, Jeffrey Weeks and Catherine Donovan

MARCUS, E. (1992) *The Male Couples's Guide: Finding a Man, Making a Home, Building a Life.* New York: Harper Perennial.

MULLER, A. (1987) *Parents Matter: Parents Relationships with Lesbian Daughters and Gay Sons.* Tallahassee, FL: Naiad Press.

NARDI, P. (1992a) 'That's what friends are for: friends as family in the lesbian and gay community', in Plummer, K. (ed.) *Modern Homosexualities: Fragments of Lesbian and Gay Experience.* London: Routledge.

NARDI, P. (1992b) 'Sex, friendship and gender roles among gay men', in Nardi, P. (ed.) *Men's Friendship.* London: Sage.

NARDI, P. and SHERROD, D. (1994) 'Friendship in the lives of gay men and lesbians', *Journal of Social and Personal Relationships,* **11**, pp. 185–99.

PLUMMER, K. (ed.) (1992) *Modern Homosexualities: Fragments of Lesbian and Gay Experience.* London: Routledge.

PLUMMER, K. (1995) *Telling Sexual Stories: Power, Change and Social Worlds.* London: Routledge.

PORTER, K. and WEEKS, J. (1990) *Between The Acts.* London: Routledge.

PRIEUR, A. (1990) 'Gay men: reasons for continued practice of unsafe sex', *AIDS Education and Prevention,* **2**, 2, pp. 110–17.

RAPHAEL, S. and ROBINSON, M. (1984) 'The older lesbian: love relationships and friendship patterns', in Darty, T. and Potter, S. (eds) *Women Identified Women.* Palo Alto, CA: Mayfield.

ROBERTS, C. and McGLONE, F. (1997) *Kinship Networks and Friendships: Attitudes and Behaviour in Britain 1986–1995.* Population and Household Change Research Programme, Research Results 3. Swindon: ESRC.

RUBIN, L. (1985) *Just Friends: The Role of Friendship in Our Lives.* New York: Harper & Row.

WEEKS, J. (1991) *Against Nature: Essays on History, Sexuality and Identity.* London: Rivers Oram Press.

WEEKS, J. (1995) *Invented Moralities: Sexual Values in an Age of Uncertainty.* Cambridge: Polity.

WEEKS, J., DONOVAN, C. and HEAPHY, B. (1996) *Families of Choice: Patterns of Non-Heterosexual Relationships. A Literature Review.* Social Science Research Papers 2, South Bank University.

WESTON, K. (1991) *Families We Choose: Lesbians, Gays, Kinship.* New York: Columbia University Press.

Chapter 6

Everyone on the Scene is so Cliquey: Are Gay Bars an Appropriate Context for a Community-Based Peer-Led Intervention?

Paul Flowers and Graham Hart

Recent conceptual approaches to HIV risk reduction (e.g. Van Campenhoudt *et al.*, 1997) have moved away from the individual focus of earlier work and have begun to address the social context of risk (Hart and Flowers, 1996; Parker, 1994). Similarly, work within the prevention field has moved beyond addressing the individual as the target of intervention and instead posits the wider social context as a more appropriate focus for risk reduction (Tawil, Verster and O'Reilly, 1995). There have been documented examples of the efficacy of such approaches among communities of gay men (Kelly *et al.*, 1991; Kelly *et al.*, 1992; Kelly *et al.*, 1997; Kegeles, Hays and Coates, 1996). Such community-level interventions are thought to be effective because they impact upon a given community's normative values. Directly changing the norms within a community seems to offer a particularly cost-effective method of intervention. One popular method of intervention which directly focuses upon norms has been the adoption of peer-led education. A major influence upon models of such peer-led education has been Rogers' (1983) diffusion-of-innovations theory. He notes that when around one-fifth of a community adopt an innovation then, as Kegeles, Hays and Coates (1996: 1129) write in relation to gay men's sexual health, 'the innovation can be conveyed through natural social networks and cause a community wide change'. This method of intervention highlights the utility of using 'popular people' or 'key opinion leaders' as the best people to endorse innovations (such as HIV risk-reducing behaviour) within a community, and 'refine behavioural norms and standards' (Kelly *et al.*, 1992: 1483).

With regard to its theoretical roots, peer education is based on the concept of normative influence. Normative influence itself occupies a rather unique position, crossing disciplinary boundaries with its merging of the social and the personal. As might be expected, it has a clear place within both social psychology and sociology. With respect to sexual behaviour, the role of normative influence has a long history with the formation of very powerful social constraints (such as morality) shaping sexual conduct (Ahlemeyer and Ludwig, 1997). Post 'sexual liberation', HIV risk reduction can be thought of as presenting people with a new code of sexual conduct; its explicitly prescriptive message renders unprotected sex the newest taboo (Guizzardi, 1997).

Many papers highlight the importance of norms affecting gay men's sexual health (Peterson *et al.*, 1992; Connell *et al.*, 1989; Cochran *et al.*, 1992, Stall *et al.*, 1990). Normative values are a central part of many psychological models which seek to predict health-related behaviour (e.g. Fishbein and Ajzen, 1975). There is a relatively long history of researching normative influence (e.g. Deutsch and Gerard, 1955) and much early social psychology focused upon this concept. Fisher (1988) has reviewed some of this work and has observed that people adhere to group norms because they fear sanctions if they are broken. Fisher also notes that similar individuals within networks are particularly effective models for implementing behavioural change. In a recent study of sexual health peer education among college students, the similarity of the peer educators was found to significantly affect their ability to become role models and shape the perception of social norms (Reeder, Pryor and Marsh, 1997).

Other paradigms address normative influence, not from the individual perspective but from a focus on the social aspects of sexual behaviour. Gagnon and Simon's (1973) work regarding sexual scripts highlights the cultural and historical specificity of sexual conduct. More microsocial approaches to understanding normative influence focus upon the interactions in which normative influence occurs (Ferrand and Snijders, 1997). According to these authors, the most effective source of normative influence within a social network is likely to be between members who have weaker social ties, as the relative costs of sanctions are less than the potential loss of a partner, or the perceived betrayal of a close friend. Ferrand and Snijders also note that overlapping of sexual networks and networks of personal friends and acquaintances are more likely to provide greater social pressure.

The commercial gay scene in non-metropolitan areas seems to present just such a situation (Flowers *et al.*, 1997). Kelly *et al.* (1991: 168) suggest that in the USA at least, gay venues in small cities 'tend to attract large, stable crowds of homosexual men and serve as the primary social setting in each city's gay community'. Thus, they may represent suitable locations for community-level peer-led interventions. The extent to which this is true of larger towns or cities remains, however, an area for further investigation. This chapter explores these issues in the context of Glasgow, Scotland.

The study reported here is part of development work contributing to the design of a community-based peer-led intervention targeting gay men using the commercial gay scene in Glasgow. The city, with its five gay bars and three gay clubs, offers opportunities for health interventions for gay men because the commercial gay scene is the focus of much social activity. And relatively speaking, Glasgow is also geographically and socially isolated from other cities, so the effect of city-specific interventions can be measured by comparing it with similar-sized cities in which no similar interventions are taking place.

In this preliminary study, we focused on the issues pertinent to community-level peer-led intervention. We adopted a multi-method approach, combining qualitative and quantitative methods to critically examine the appropriateness of basing such an intervention in the commercial gay scene. Our two central research aims were, firstly, to examine the feasibility of using the commercial gay scene in Glasgow as a place within which to access large numbers of gay men; and secondly, to examine the social context of the gay scene as an appropriate forum for community-based peer-led intervention. We found that Glasgow's commercial gay scene does provide an excellent source of access to gay men and thus would seem, on initial consideration, to provide an ideal environment for a gay men's peer-led intervention. However, in contrast to the optimism generated by our quantitative findings, qualitative research indicated a profound fragmentation of gay 'community' and gay identity; and the resulting disparity seriously called into question the appropriateness of recruiting other gay men as 'peers', simply because they were also on the scene. In our conclusion we propose a resolution of this dilemma which may have implications for future community-based peer-led interventions.

Methods

This study employed a variety of methods: participant observation, self-completed questionnaires within a survey, and individual in-depth interviews. Although the combination of different methods was an integral part of the research design, only a brief description of each is presented here.

Participant Observation

Throughout the study we had an ongoing commitment to participant observation. Particular details of the social dynamics of the scene were supplemented with an intense one-week census period in which the exact number of men using each venue was recorded at two separate time periods each evening (early and late). This sought to determine the feasibility of the sexual behaviour survey (see below) and the feasibility of a peer-led community-level intervention.

Survey

A short questionnaire was developed requesting information concerning demographics (postcode, age, socioeconomic class), sexually transmitted infections (STIs), use of the commercial gay scene, perceptions of a safer-sex culture and recent sexual behaviour. Over a four-week period, 14 visits were made to each of the five commercial gay bars in Glasgow city centre (70 visits in all). The results of this survey were analyzed using SPSS (Hart *et al.*, forthcoming). Analyses were concerned to assess the need for peer-led community-level intervention (i.e. high levels of reported HIV risk behaviour), and to examine associations between the use of the commercial gay scene and sexual health behaviours.

In-depth Interviews

Twenty individual interviews were conducted with a range of gay men. Men were interviewed by either a gay male interviewer or a heterosexual female interviewer. These men were contacted through a combination of methods: cold contacts within bars, snowballing from existing contacts, and participation in focus groups. A wide range of men were interviewed, reflecting the variety of men who use the commercial gay scene. The interviews covered three broad subject areas: the commercial gay scene, relationships and sexual activity. They focused upon participants' experiences and perspectives and, as such, were mostly structured by the participant's own disclosures. Interviews were recorded on audio cassette then transcribed verbatim. We used interpretative phenomenological analysis (Smith, Flowers and Osborne, 1997) to analyse transcripts, using a combination of manual coding and NUD.IST software.

The process of analysis involved several steps. In order to engage with the participants' view of their world, we attempted to suspend any preconceived ideas relating to the commercial gay scene and gay men's sexual health. Following this, each transcript was analysed for emergent themes; these were identified by the recurrence of key words, phrases or understandings. After repeating the process with each individual transcript, recurrent themes were listed which reflected shared understandings across different interviews. The resulting analysis reflects the underlying ways in which men connect the commercial gay scene to other aspects of their lives.

Findings

It is beyond the scope of this chapter to report the full results of each of the methods used. Instead, we will address our two central research questions: the extent to which it is feasible to use the commercial gay scene in Glasgow as a place within which to access large numbers of gay men; and whether the social context of the gay scene is an appropriate setting for community-based peer-led interventions.

Table 6.1   Frequency of visits to the gay scene in Glasgow

Frequency of visits to the scene	Number of men
4–5 times per week	191 (16%)
1–2 per week	495 (40%)
2–3 times per month	383 (31%)
Rarely	155 (13%)

Participant Observation

The spatial organization of Glasgow's commercial gay scene is important in understanding the movement of gay men between bars. Each venue is positioned within the city centre, with a five-minute walk separating most of the five gay bars; two mixed bars were excluded from both the census and the survey because of their combined heterosexual and gay clientele.

In addressing the first research question (feasibility of access), the census enumerated the number of gay men attending the five commercial gay bars within a one-week period at two distinct time periods (early evening and late evening). The resulting figure ($n = 2,616$) is likely to overestimate the total number of men present because many would have been double-counted within any given evening and/or across evenings. However, even assuming strict double counting, with approximately 1,300 men attending the commercial scene on a weekly basis, we felt that the bars represent a feasible context for approaching large numbers of gay men. Participant observation indicated that only when specific events (karaoke or quiz nights) were taking place did there appear to be potential difficulties with audibility or gaining the attention of men within the bars.

Survey

The potential of the bar scene to permit contact with large numbers of gay men was proven by the survey itself. Of all men approached and asked to complete a self-administered questionnaire, 77 per cent agreed to do so, providing a sample of 1,245 men. Table 6.1 describes the frequency of visits to the commercial gay scene. Most of the men were regular attenders, with 56 per cent visiting the bars more than once per week. The sample was typical of other recent studies of British gay men (Hart *et al.*, 1993; Davies *et al.*, 1993) in that approximately one-third reported having engaged in unprotected anal intercourse within the previous year.

Chi-squared tests were conducted to assess the association between the frequency of visits to the gay scene and other variables. No significant associations were found between frequency of visits to the gay scene and socioeconomic class, perceptions of a safer sex culture, HIV risk-related behaviour – defined as any unprotected anal intercourse (UAI) in the preceding year – frequency of condom use, sexually transmitted diseases in the last year, level of highest qualification, employment status or age. However, significant associations were found between frequency of visits to the gay scene and reports of ever having had an STI (p < .03). Men who used the scene most often reported higher numbers of sexual partners within the last month (p < .00001) and also higher numbers of anal penetrative partners (p < .007) within the last month. With regard to the preceding year, men who visited the scene most often reported higher numbers of sexual partners (p < .00001) and higher numbers of anal penetrative partners (p < .00005). Thus, a higher frequency of visits to the scene was significantly associated with relatively high levels of sexual activity. No significant associations were found, however, between scene use and number of partners with whom unprotected anal sex took place.

Differences between the five bars were also examined. Participant observation had shown that each venue had its own distinct 'regulars' but also that significant numbers of men travelled from one bar to the other throughout the evening, reaping the benefits of each venue's 'happy hour', for example. While there were no differences between the five bars in terms of a wide range of variables, including HIV risk-related behaviour, there were significant differences between the bars in terms of age (p < .00001), men's educational qualifications (p < .05) and reported sexually transmitted infections within the previous year (p < .01).

In-depth Interviews

During the individual in-depth interviews, men often talked about the commercial gay scene. They described at length the differences between the bars and the changing clientele over the nights of the week, and they presented a range of reasons as to why and how men use the scene. Many men talked of the scene in similar terms, and such representations reappeared throughout the interviews. A frequent comment related to men's apparent disenchantment with the 'scene'; it was repeatedly described as 'superficial'. However, as one participant commented, and we uncovered data which supported this view, 'A lot of people think of it as shallow. I don't see it as shallow. I think it is quite complicated, quite deep.'

It is around this simple opposition, between assumed simplicity and, as we shall see, an emerging complexity, that this analysis examines the scene as a potential social context for community-based peer-led intervention. Within the literature, it often seems that one city's gay scene is interchangeable with another's (Kelly *et al.*, 1992), one gay bar is much like another and that one gay community is much like another (Asthana and Oostvogels, 1996). It is implicitly assumed that gay men, and particularly gay men using the scene, constitute a homogeneous group. It is in opposition to this unitary understanding that we can contrast our interpretation of the accounts of the men who took part in this study.

In examining the gay scene at one level, peer education within gay bars seems relatively straightforward. For example, a shared gay identity could represent a suitable level of conceptualizing gay men's 'peers', and interactions between gay men *per se* would maximize the affects of social influence. However, when men spoke of their experiences on the scene, the salience of shared gay identity was lost and a host of other identities and social dynamics emerged as crucial in understanding social interactions. As one participant commented, 'You know, the only thing that brings all these people under the one roof is the fact that they are all gay and probably 85 per cent of them are trying to get laid.' This suggests there is some commonality among men found in gay bars; they share a desire for sex with other men. However, this is certainly not grounds to assume that they have anything else in common.

Three key recurrent themes were identified which illustrate some of the complexity of social interactions within the commercial gay scene and also highlight the importance of normative influence: (i) the scene as parochial and familiar, (ii) gossip as a mechanism for individual control and (iii) group dynamics and social control.

The Scene as Parochial and Familiar

Many men talked of the scene in terms of its small size, the scene in Glasgow representing a relatively closed social environment. Although each bar had a distinct group of regular users, most also attracted a crowd of mobile men visiting many bars within each evening. In this situation, people become readily identifiable to one another. As one participant describes it:

The scene is very small, everybody knows everyone, and everyone knows each other's business. (Participant S)

Many men talked of the scene being 'boring', filled with the 'same old faces' and as essentially predictable. Newcomers to the scene could easily be identified and were described as 'fresh meat'. In this environment, familiar faces were sometimes given names and identities. As the following extract shows:

I mean there's like, there's two guys I know actually who are called Cagney and Lacey, I think its because they go about in their car all the time, pick people up then take them away. (S)

This illustrates the perceived incestuous nature of the commercial gay scene in Glasgow. However, it was not only individuals who were recognizable, but also distinct social groupings. Some men described the scene as being tribal, or based around clans or, as the next extract shows, families.

> There is always wee groups. I suppose you get to know people and what happens is, like it is wee families, like he's my pal and that. (J)

These social groupings are important because they fragment the uniformity of the scene. Interactions between gay men are patterned according to both relations between groups and between individuals within groups. Many of these groups had distinct names, such as neds, schemies and giros[1]; other names are sad old queens, the young crowd, workies, the in-crowd, the beautiful people, the top lot. Individual behaviour is understood as shaped by such group membership; as one self-identified 'professional' gay man commented, regarding imagined difficulties in our recruitment of non-professional men into this study:

> They are the screaming hairdressers with hard candy nail polish and the satin blouses and all the rest of it. All the really camp queens, and there is a lot of them on the Glasgow scene. You will never get them to come and you will never get these muscle Marys to come – they are too busy at the gym or whatever. The ones with the big bodies that guarantee a small dick and they walk around with their cropped haircuts. (K)

Among gay men in Glasgow, it appears that group membership is pivotal in understanding relations between individual gay men. Among men using the scene regularly, there was a hierarchy of groups with 'the top lot' being the best and the 'schemies' being positioned, as one respondent described it, at the 'lower end of the market'. As the following extract describes them:

> Neds and schemies are just sort of, I don't know how, sorry there's not a really nice way of putting this, they're just the scum really, guaranteed they're probably off spending money on drugs, getting absolutely drunk whenever they go out, causing trouble most of the time. They're the ones like that have the fake fabulous clothes, the labels sewn on in a hurry. (T)

In summary, we can understand the gay scene in Glasgow as being perceived as small, both in terms of the number of people and the number of possible venues. This situation facilitates a set of dynamics in which the same people repeatedly meet each other and the people who use the scene are thought of as falling into distinct types of people or social groupings.

Gossip and Control

All the men who took part in this study commented on the 'bitchy' nature of the scene, and the 'attitude' of people therein. Bitchiness often related to people's group membership, or factors which related to it, e.g. their appearance, clothing or hairstyle. Bitchiness also directly addressed individuals in terms of their reputation, penis size, their HIV status, sexual performance and their behaviour. Many men talked of the two-faced nature of the scene, e.g. the public presentation of friendliness and the often vicious conversation reported in private. As the following extract shows:

> People in the gay scene are so back-stabbing. I've been in somebody's company like, and it is the same anywhere, more so on the gay scene. You are in a group and there is a guy joining us and then the guy walks away and they go like, 'He's a fucking whore. He got shagged by so and so. 'He is this and he is that. (S)

This excerpt shows the centrality of sexual reputation in scene gossip. As the following quote suggests, such reputational gossip not only addresses particular individuals but also their sexual partners and their reputations:

> Oh you find out, gossip. Somebody told somebody, somebody told somebody else, it gets spread throughout the bar, everybody gets a different version of it and I mean it's like, 'You got crabs last week Ha-ha! And we all know who you got it from as well and you shouldn't be surprised because he's been around the block more than once.' (S)

Gossip within the scene is capable of gathering a momentum of its own. This discourse is important because of the impact it has on individual's behaviour. 'Bitchiness' too can be thought of as a method of control in the way it provides a pervasive sense of surveillance which tacitly shapes people's behaviour:

> You're being watched, everything you do, so if you're seen with a different person, not necessarily sleeping with them, a different night, you're like the gossip of the scene. (S)

Because of these pressures many men talked about the importance of self-presentation, in terms of 'image' and of putting on 'fronts':

> I mean image is such a big thing when you go up to the scene, doing this, doing that, wearing this, wearing that. (S)

There are injunctive social norms, therefore, which structure interactions upon the gay scene. As some of the extracts have indicated, the content of these prescriptions ranges from choice of sexual partner to the labelling of designer clothes. What emerges is a powerful sense of normative influence at work. Men feel constrained by an awareness of the 'public' forum which gay bars present. Indeed, fear for one's own reputation can directly affect one's behaviour:

> And they don't want to make a move because you doesn't want to be seen as a cow or a slut, right. There is always two-faced shit you know. Like I've been with him, I fucked him and he was a lousy shag and he's got a small dick, and he's got a tight arse and all this sort of shit. All that crap goes on. (S)

In summary it appears there are very powerful normative influences at work between gay men on the scene. Bitchiness and gossip provide a backdrop against which public behaviour can be measured. Men feel constrained by normative expectations of other gay men visiting the gay bars.

Group Dynamics and Control

The last theme focused upon an individual perspective of the power of 'attitude' and gossip in affecting gay men on the scene in Glasgow. However, it is also interesting to focus upon the relationship between such gossip and the group structure of the gay scene in Glasgow. Several men actually talked of 'social climbing' between groups; for example, the participant below recounted a conversation with someone he understood to belong to the 'top lot':

> He told me at one point that I could do very well for myself on the scene and why do you hang about with that bunch of losers. They are not losers, they are my friends, I know these people. (K)

The same participant went on to talk about how group membership created a barrier between gay men. He described how difficult it would be for any discussion to occur between the 'in-crowd' and the 'cruising' crowd:

K I honestly don't think one of the younger in-crowd would give the older, 'older' is the wrong word but, one of the 'cruising' crowd the time of day. I think there's a certain disparagement, they're looked down upon by the younger in-crowd.
P What kind of things would they say about them?
K Er various phrases – slappers, tosspots.
P What is a tosspot and what is a slapper?
K (laughs) Er – anyone who is not part of your crowd.

Here again, we can see the importance of sexual reputation, with the participant's ironic comment 'anyone who is not part of your crowd' highlighting the functional aspect of reputational slander in delineating group membership.

Peer group pressure also influences partner choice, with the development of a relationship being influenced by group membership:

P   Why would they get slagged off?
S   Because they've been seen to be getting off with somebody that's not up to their standards, or their friend's standards. I found that a lot as well, your friends kind of say, 'He's not very nice, what are you doing with him?' Then you're forced into going with a certain person; if your friends don't like them that's it, you can't. You feel as if you have to kind of dump them.

Some men talked about how social interactions were shaped by group membership, for example, who would or would not talk to whom. Age and clothing differences emerged as important. The previous quote suggested that there is some notion of a 'right' kind of sexual partner for a group member to find attractive and want a relationship with. The extract below indicates how problematic some of these dynamics can be:

You take it to the extent where anyone that you don't fancy, is not attractive in your eyes, anyone you are not interested in being attracted to you, you alienate them, like you blank them, you won't speak to them? That takes it too far.

We have outlined the potential difficulties of assuming that gay men are equally likely to talk to each other; interactions are patterned according to group membership and perceived peer surveillance. Individual behaviour is constrained by peer approval. Dress, hairstyle, conversation and partner choice were all clearly reported to be shaped by normative influence. Normative values relating to sexual health also emerge as important. However, when they were reported they focused largely upon reputation as identifying certain individuals as vectors of disease (e.g. carrying crabs). We were surprised that we did not find evidence of explicit injunctions relating to HIV risk-related behaviour. No one talked of 'bitchiness' directly relating to a lack of condom use, for example. Where HIV was discussed, it again related to given individuals as possible sources of infection rather than illustrating an acceptance of the universal threat of HIV resulting from the occurrence of unprotected anal sex.

The results of the survey (i.e. around one-third of men reporting some UAI) indicated that unprotected sex occurs, and they suggest the limited extent to which safer sex values are an integral part of the bar culture of gay men in Glasgow. The absence of gossip relating to condom use suggests that safer sex is not a key element in the normative discourse of gay men in the city, unlike other more public aspects of gay lifestyle (self-presentation, fashion, etc.)

Discussion

Findings from this preliminary study suggest that in some ways Glasgow's commercial gay scene renders it a suitable environment in which to conduct peer-led education. Large numbers of men attend a limited number of bars at least once a week, and many make multiple visits. Most of the bars are no more than five minutes walk from each other, and this spatial propinquity means that peer educators could easily access and work in several different bars during the course of an evening, and speak to many different men.

Yet questions arise as to the appropriateness and nature of any peer education that can take place in these settings. The effects of normative influence are attenuated by perceived 'dissimilarity' between peers (Fisher, 1988; Reeder, Pryor and Harsh, 1997). It is clear from recent studies that gay men do not constitute a homogeneous group, not only in terms of their sexual behaviour (Hart *et al.*, 1993; Davies *et al.*, 1993) but also socially and demographically (Hope and McArthur, 1998). Will men consider those who approach them to be truly their 'peers', or will they perceive them as above, below or simply from a different social stratum? Will they ignore people who are not recognized as being of their own social group? The data from our qualitative interviews suggests the picture is complex, as it is apparent that the gay scene is constituted not only of men differentiated by social class and education, but also of a nexus of relatively discrete social networks of known individuals and couples who have been attributed certain identifying features – features considered to be more or less distinct from their own microsocial unit of current attachment. Can the neds, schemies and giros interact with the beautiful people or the top lot, and does each have any influence or the potential to have any impact upon the others' views and behaviours?

Although the analysis of the in-depth interviews offers a rather bleak picture of the social life of Glasgow's gay scene – social relations marked by others' prescriptions over choice of friendship group, partner and even cloth-ing – what this does highlight is the everyday reality and potency of normative injunctions for men on the scene. 'Bitchiness' and gossip are a key part of this social world, and these (private and personal) discourses serve as mechanisms for surveillance and control over (public) behaviour. Yet there lies within these discourses and social relations the potential for a very focused form of peer education involving the use of social-network-specific, indigenous outreach workers. These would need to be gay men and women (regardless of sexuality) who use the gay scene in Glasgow and are recruited from within, rather than outside, the social networks that constitute the scene. Coming from a position of security and trust within the identified microsocial units that are evident to many who visit the scene, it would be their task to privilege a discourse of safer sex and positive sexual health to others of their own social background and shared structural and cultural location. This would be done in the context of the reality of the constraints and opportunities afforded by their daily lives and with the full knowledge of the men to whom they are talking. Exploiting the key role of normative injunctions regarding selection of friends, partners, and group membership, the aim should be to establish HIV risk-reducing behaviour as a central normative value, using cultural sensitivity and experience to communicate these messages effectively. Safer sex could thereby become one more normative injunction, along with friendship or dress. Normative injunctions are clearly effective within gay bars, and so the aim is to make sexual health normatively pre-emptive in the domain of sex and sexuality.

With respect to this aim, one further issue must be to address the difference between 'public' and 'private' behaviour. Since sexual behaviour occurs in Glasgow beyond the public and overtly social arena of the gay bars, it remains a challenge to ensure that the gap between what is perceived as socially acceptable and what actually takes place is narrowed.

Many problems associated with peer education have arisen because of the absence of any clear consensus as to what constitutes peer education, its theoretical underpinnings and the parameters of effectiveness (Milburn, 1995). One particular issue has been that the impact of peer education is often greatest on peer educators themselves rather than on their target populations. It is unclear how a focus on such 'empowerment', though valuable in its own right, can help implement change beyond those directly involved in such peer education training. However, we believe the form that peer education in Glasgow should take could be derived from the research we have conducted on the scene, being grounded in the data generated through qualitative interviews. Such an approach would also be theoretically informed by a literature which both describes the normative mechanisms to be employed by individual peers, and the community-wide effect it is intended to achieve through the diffusion of innovation. It is clear that unitary notions of a 'gay community' or 'gay identity' are quite inappropriate to this context, and it is only by identifying and working with the social relations which exist between people on the gay scene in a city such as Glasgow that it will be possible to realize the full potential of social-network-specific, indigenous outreach workers.

Note

1 Neds can be thought of as young thugs; the name has connotations of antisocial behaviour. Schemies are people living in council estates or hous-

ing schemes. Giros are named after their sporadic visits to the scene, visits which depend on the arrival of their unemployment benefit.

References

AHLEMEYER, H.W. and LUDWIG, D. (1997) 'Norms of communication and communication as a norm in the intimate social system', in Van Campenhoudt, L., Cohen, M., Guizzardi, G. and Hausser, D. (eds) *Sexual Interactions and HIV Risk: New Conceptual Perspectives in European Research*. London: Taylor & Francis.

ASTHANA, S. and OOSTVOGELS, R. (1996) 'Community participation in HIV prevention: problems and prospects for community-based strategies among female sex workers in Madras', *Social Science and Medicine*, **43**, pp. 133–48.

COCHRAN, S., MAYS, V.M., CLARETTA, J., CARUSO, C. and MALLON, D. (1992) 'Efficacy of the theory of reasoned action in predicting AIDS-related sexual risk-reduction among gay men', *Journal of Applied Social Psychology*, **22**, pp. 1481–1501.

CONNELL, R.W., CRAWFORD, J., KIPPAX, S., DOWSETT, G.W., BAXTER, D., WATSON, L. and BERG, R. (1989) 'Facing the epidemic: changes in the sexual lives of gay and bisexual men in Australia and their implications for AIDS prevention strategies', *Social Problems*, **36**, pp. 384–402.

DAVIES, P., HICKSON, F., WEATHERBURN, P. and HUNT, A. (1993) *Sex, Gay Men and AIDS*. London: Falmer Press.

DEUTSCH, M. and GERARD, H.B. (1955) 'A study of normative and informational social influences on individual judgement', *Journal of Abnormal and Social Psychology*, **51**, pp. 629–36.

FERRAND, A. and SNIJDERS, T. (1997) 'Social networks and normative tensions', in Van Campenhoudt, L., Cohen, M., Guizzardi, G. and Hausser, D. (eds) *Sexual Interactions and HIV Risk: New Conceptual Perspectives in European Research*. London: Taylor & Francis.

FISHBEIN, M. and AJZEN, I. (1975) *Belief, Attitude, Intent and Behaviour: An Introduction to Theory and Research*. Reading, MA: Addison-Wesley.

FISHER, J.D. (1988) 'Possible effects of reference group-based social influence on AIDS-risk behaviour and AIDS prevention', *American Psychologist*, **43**, pp. 914–20.

FLOWERS, P., SMITH, J.A., SHEERAN, P. and BEAIL, N. (1997). 'Identities and gay men's sexual decision making', in Aggleton, P., Davies, P. and Hart, G. (eds) *AIDS: Activism and Alliances*. London: Taylor & Francis.

GAGNON, J.H. and SIMON, W. (1973). *Sexual Conduct: The Social Sources of Human Sexuality*. London: Hutchinson.

GUIZZARDI, G. (1997) 'Norms of relationship and normative tensions', in Van Campenhoudt, L., Cohen, M., Guizzardi, G. and Hausser, D (eds) *Sexual*

Interactions and HIV Risk: New Conceptual Perspectives in European Research. London: Taylor & Francis.

HART, G. and FLOWERS, P. (1996) A survey of gay men's sexual behaviour in Glasgow. Unpublished paper, Medical Sociology Unit, Glasgow.

HART, G., FLOWERS, P., DER, G. and FRANKIS, J. (in press) 'Gay men's HIV-related sexual risk behaviour in Scotland', *Sexually Transmitted Infections.*

HART, G.J., DAWSON, J., FITZPATRICK, R.M., BOULTON, M., MCLEAN, J., BROOKES, M. and PARRY, J.V. (1993) 'Risk behaviour, anti-HIV and anti-hepatitis B core prevalence in clinic and non-clinic samples of gay men in England, 1991–1992', *AIDS*, **7**, pp. 863–69.

HOPE, V.D. and MACARTHUR, C. (1998) 'Safer sex and social class: findings from a study of men using the 'gay scene' in the West Midlands region of the United Kingdom', *AIDS Care*, **10**, pp. 81–88.

KEGELES, S.M., HAYS, R.B. and COATES, T.J. (1996) 'The Mpowerment Project: a community-level HIV prevention intervention for young gay men', *American Journal of Public Health*, **86**, pp. 1129–36.

KELLY, J.A., ST LAWRENCE, J.S., DIAZ, Y.E., STEVENSON, L.Y., HAUTH, A.C., BRASFIELD, T.L., KALICHMAN, S.C., SMITH, J.E. and ANDREW, M.E. (1991) 'HIV risk behaviour reduction following intervention with key opinion leaders of population: an experimental analysis', *American Journal of Public Health*, **81**, pp. 168–71.

KELLY, J.A., ST LAWRENCE, J.S., STEVENSON, L.Y., HAUTH, A.C., KALICHMAN, S.C., DIAZ, Y.E., BRASFIELD, T.L., KOOB, J.J. and MORGAN, M.G. (1992) 'Community AIDS/HIV risk reduction: the effects of endorsements by popular people in three cities', *American Journal of Public Health*, **82**, pp. 1483–89.

KELLY, J.A., MURPHY, D.A., SIKKEMA, K.S., MCAULIFFE, T.L., ROFFMAN, R.A., SOLOMON, L.J., WINETT, R.A., KALICHMAN, S.C. and the COMMUNITY HIV PREVENTION RESEARCH COLLABORATIVE (1997) 'Randomised, controlled, community-level HIV prevention intervention for sexual-risk behaviour among homosexual men in US cities', *Lancet*, **350**, 1500–1505.

MILBURN, K. (1995) 'A critical review of peer education with young people with special reference to sexual health', *Health Education Research*, **10**, pp. 407–20.

PARKER, R.G. (1994) 'Sexual cultures, HIV transmission, and AIDS prevention', *AIDS*, **8**, pp. S309–14.

PETERSON, J.L., COATES, T.J., CATANIA, J.A., MIDDLETON, L., HILLIARD, B. and HEARST, N. (1992) 'High risk sexual behaviour and condom use among gay and bisexual African-American men', *American Journal of Public Health*, **82**, pp. 1490–94.

REEDER, G.D., PRYOR, J.B. and HARSH, L. (1997) 'Activity and similarity in safer sex workshops led by peer educators', *AIDS Education and Prevention*, **9**, suppl. A, pp. 77–89.

ROGERS, E.M. (1983) *Diffusion of Innovations*. New York: Free Press.

SMITH, J.A., FLOWERS, P. and OSBORNE, M. (1997) 'Interpretative phenomenological analysis and the psychology of health and illness', in Yardley, L. (ed.) *The Material Discourses of Health and Illness*. London: Routledge.

STALL, R., EKSTRAND, M., POLLACK, L., McKUSICK, L. and COATES, T.J. (1990) 'Relapse from safer sex: the next challenge for AIDS prevention efforts', *Journal of the Acquired Immune Deficiency Syndromes*, **3**, pp. 1181–87.

TAWIL, O., VERSTER, A. and O'REILLY, K.R. (1995) 'Enabling approaches for HIV/AIDS prevention – can we modify the environment and minimise the risk', *AIDS*, **9**, pp. 1299–1306.

VAN CAMPENHOUDT, L., COHEN, M., GUIZZARDI, G. and HAUSSER, D. (1997) *Sexual Interactions and HIV Risk*. London: Taylor & Francis.

Chapter 7

Coming Together: Social Networks of Gay Men and HIV Prevention

Kevin Eisenstadt and Philip Gatter

It has long been argued that success in HIV prevention depends on an under-standing of the social contexts and histories in which sexual lives are developed (e.g. Altman, 1986; Dowsett *et al.*, 1992; Watney, 1993; Gatter, 1995). Sociologists such as Hart and Boulton have argued that a fuller account of social context is required for understanding properly how and why sexual risks are taken, and that we need to aim for 'the development of a sociology of risk that can account for and explain risk in terms of community membership and social structural location' (Hart and Boulton, 1995: 56). The purpose of such work is to transcend the limitations of earlier enquiry into sexual risk which focused on individual decision making within a psychological or social psychological framework. In particular, Hart and Boulton argue that we need a less abstract treatment of social variables:

> In [psychological and social psychological schemas] ... socio-economic location, age and ethnicity are simply descriptive variables included with others in statistical analyses rather than what they really are – shorthand terms for complex and multi-dimensional social processes and experiences. (Hart and Boulton, 1995: 57)

In line with this perspective, attention has turned to an operational concept of gay community as it may influence knowledge, attitudes, and risk behaviours relating to HIV. Notable analyses of the significance of gay community and degrees of gay community attachment have come from Australia, particularly in the work of Dennis Altman, Susan Kippax, Bob Connell and Gary Dowsett (Altman, 1994; Kippax *et al.* 1993). Indeed, a sophisticated understanding of the role of community must inform HIV prevention strategies:

> It is clear we need a more complex understanding of the social and sexual structuring of communities, of how each community operates, what its cultural rituals, processes and resources are, and situate the local epidemic at the heart of that understanding, if we are to mobilise communities more effectively in HIV/AIDS programmes. (Dowsett and McInnes, 1996: 3)

In recent work, Dowsett and McInnes have explored the differences between gay communities in Sydney and Adelaide using critical ethnography,[1] finding that Sydney had a large gay community focused on a particular area of the city (Oxford Street), and associated with an open gay lifestyle. Adelaide in contrast had no distinct gay locale, but gay life here depended instead on friendship circles and loose social networks. These contrasting situations have implications for how sexual health promotion might best be attempted. Such differences also suggest that in a metropolis the size of London assumptions of homogeneity are unwise.

There remains, we would argue, another valid perspective useful in framing social analyses of sexual identities, but one which has been little used. Between the poles of identity-based community and individual sexual behaviour lies a middle ground of what could be termed the socialized sexuality[2] of individuals. Socialized sexualities can include on the one hand dyadic relationships involving sex, and on the other involvement in political, social and community groupings which grow out of more local, intimate attachments. Sexualities are, of course, developed through time, and may be connected with residential migration between and within different communities (Bell and Valentine, 1995; Weston, 1995). We might reasonably treat migration as a distinct phenomenon, since physical relocation will involve (to varying degrees) the breaking and making of social networks. It is a significant change, though, since as we shall discuss, migration is not necessarily a fully planned and rationalized event at the time. We must also pay attention to the variety of factors encouraging migration; sexuality, minority sexuality in this case, may logically only be one factor, and we must analyse the relations between these different influences.

In this chapter we will consider socialized sexualities with a focus on migration to London, residence within the city, and the spatial and affective dimensions of social networks (where socializing occurs and with which kinds of people). In so doing, we will give less attention to the specifically sexual dimension of specifically gay socializing. Our data on sexual behaviours is presented elsewhere (Annetts, Eisenstadt and Gatter, 1996), but we would argue that the social data is just as valuable in understanding the contexts within which health promotion is attempted. Social networks often frame sexual tastes and opportunities. Communities premised on sexuality will clearly encompass closely intertwined social and sexual experiences, but we suggest that a preoccupation with the sexual can, ironically, obscure a more properly social understanding of HIV/AIDS. The sociology proposed by Hart and Boulton is, after all, a sociology of *risk* with the sexual behaviour bearing risk dominating the direction and focus of analysis, although this is understandable in the context of HIV prevention. In other work there has also been a tendency to elide the social and sexual aspects of being gay which, at least on analytical grounds, is not acceptable. Dowsett and McInnes, for example, find it easy to state that they are describing the structure of social (*and therefore sexual*) relations in these communities (Sydney and Adelaide). (Dowsett and McInnes, 1996: 2; emphasis added)

Here we hope to balance a preoccupation with the sexual by focusing more on the social. This may also be useful in thinking about future health promotion strategies. Sexual networks, for example, have already been used as access points for prevention. Gay Men Fighting AIDS (GMFA) has used them when working in public sex environments (PSEs) in London such as Hampstead Heath. Finally, we want to add to existing literature on the life histories and migration of gay men and lesbians in and to Britain, (Brighton Ourstory Project, 1992; Cant, 1997) and to recent sociological work on the globalization of sexual identities (e.g. Altman, 1997; Bao, 1997; Carrilo, 1997; Tan, 1995).

The data discussed here is specific to an area of London which at first sight may seem parochial. We would argue that the material is of interest in itself, as well as in suggesting directions for further research on sexual identities and communities. First, many studies of gay communities have been located in the USA, and focus on the establishment of gay ghettos and processes of gentrification (Castells, 1983; Herdt, 1992; Levine, 1979). Second, where the UK is concerned, it is Soho in central London which has been most written about. Mort (1996), for example, discussed Soho as a gay-coded space in *Cultures of Consumption*. By way of contrast, our research concerns parts of south London, which is as much a place where gay men live as socialize. Third, Plummer, in his afterword to a recent collection on social perspectives in lesbian and gay studies (Nardi and Schneider, 1998) decries the lack of good empirical sociological research on lesbian and gay identity and community. He identifies a preponderance of textual analysis (linked to postmodernism) and cultural studies (of which Mort's book is one example), and states:

I do not know of a single published ethnography of any aspect of London's lesbian/gay scene. (Plummer, 1998: 612)

We hope this chapter may go some way to filling the gap.

The data presented here was collected in a research project funded by Lambeth, Southwark and Lewisham Health Authority (LSL), and entitled the *Gay and Bisexual Men's HIV Prevention Service Review and Social Mapping Project*. This project aimed to collect information on current service provision and delineate the local population of gay and bisexual men as a resource for developing the medium- to long-term health promotion commissioning strategy of LSL. In practice, data collection took place almost exclusively from self-identifying gay men, and the following analysis refers specifically to this group of respondents.

The project took place in two stages. Work began with a questionnaire survey which collected basic social and sexual data from a group of 570 men (accessed via service providers, gay organization mailing lists, snowballing and personal contacts) most of whom were resident in LSL. From this survey, 15 individuals were selected purposively, covering a range of variables (age, ethnic origin, residence, time spent in London) and interviewed in depth about their social and sexual lives.

Structurally our material is presented in terms of the histories of socialized sexualities. We examine first how and why our interviewees moved to London. Then we look at how they have moved once in the city, paying attention to the significance of being gay for choices over where to live. We then discuss gay social infrastructure, considering which venues people use and why, according to context and personal history. Wider identifications are then considered, including gay community involvement and the structuring of networks around influences such as ethnicity. Finally, we consider the significance of our data in the context of HIV prevention.

Some of what we have to say has been stated anecdotally elsewhere. We believe that the systematic collection of social data, while not necessarily in tension with the 'common knowledge' of the gay population, brings greater depth and nuancing to our understanding of the gay social world. Identifications, choices about where to live and the complexities of socializing suggest that London is something more than a 'gay magnet', while undeniably being one.

Migration to London

In their report on gay men's social and sexual mobility in London, Kelley, Pebody and Scott (1996) assert that London exerts a major migratory pull on gay men. In their sample of 1,001 men recruited from a wide variety of gay commercial venues across London, 77.1 per cent currently resident in London had not grown up there but had moved to the capital as adults. Similarly, in our own questionnaire sample of 570 men, 70 per cent were born outside London (Annetts, Eisenstadt and Gatter, 1996).[3] These findings are in line with those from larger quantitative studies, such as NATSAL (Johnson *et al.*, 1994) in the UK and NHSLS (Michael *et al.*, 1994) in the USA. Johnson *et al.* found that some 12 per cent of all men in greater London reported same-sex sexual contact during their lifetimes, compared with 6.1 per cent for the UK as a whole. In the USA, 9 per cent of men in the 12 largest cities identified themselves as gay; in rural areas fewer than 1 per cent did so.[4] If homosexual contact over the past five years only is considered (which is taken as a proxy of being currently homosexually active) then the contrast between London and elsewhere in the UK is even greater, with 8.6 per cent responding positively in inner London compared to 1.4 per cent outside the capital.

In our study we only interviewed gay men, so we are not in a position to make direct comparisons with other people's reasons for migration to London. But there is, however, quantified data from NATSAL which supports the view that in-migration to London by gay men is significantly greater than for other sections of the population:

> The concentration of those reporting homosexual experience in the capital is most striking. . . . Table 7.6 shows that men and women who report a homosexual partner in the past 5 years are far more likely to have moved to live in London than are those who do not, and this difference is not apparent for migration elsewhere in Britain. (Johnson *et al.*, 1994: 195)

While care must be taken in equating same-sex activity with 'being' a gay man or lesbian, these findings do support the view that migration, especially to metropolitan areas, is a key factor accounting for the population distribution of gay men. Various reasons have been suggested for this, including the opportunity for more social and sexual contact with other members of a minority, and the relative anonymity of the big city for a stigmatized population (Coxon, 1985; Johnson *et al.*, 1994). But to date, these rationales are largely based on speculation and anecdotal evidence. The reasons why individuals move, both to and within cities, are clearly qualitative questions, and we explored these questions via in-depth interviews. Such a small number of respondents cannot be taken as statistically representative of any group, but the interviews contain rich accounts of the mobility patterns and the reasons underlying them. They offer important insight into the way in which migration, particularly sexual migration, is conceptualized.[5] In the section on migration which follows, all quotations and discussion derive from our interview data.

Adult International Migration

To say that interviewees moved to London to lead a gay lifestyle would be an oversimplification, and plainly inaccurate in some cases. This is most notably true for those who came to London in adulthood from outside the UK. Being gay was a significant factor in migration for some, but was not necessarily the dominant concern in choosing London. Thus interviewees from the Caribbean and Brazil came to London in the hope of acquiring recognized educational qualifications. One of these two was only 18 at the time of immigration, and was not yet sure of his sexual orientation. The other had been homosexually active in his community of origin but with the restriction that, as an unmarried man, he was expected to continue living with his parents, and to live with another man in an openly gay relationship would have been virtually unthinkable:

> You have to get married to leave the house. They see like if you are leaving the house it's because you're not happy so you don't even

have any need to talk to us any more, that's how they react. So we have to stay living with our parents so we can't have boyfriends. So that's why everyone leave the country, so I mean that's why I live my gay life the way I want here. I couldn't live like that in Brazil at all. My mother would not accept. If I go back to Brazil I have to live with her.

This same interviewee described how Brazilians like himself tend to migrate to one of the major American cities since the USA is closer and cheaper to get to than England. He had also been told of the infamous emotional coldness and conservatism of the English. The choice of London was for him almost accidental. He had just finished a relationship in difficult circumstances and

it was time to have a break from everything. Family, work, college, I said, 'Ah, I've got to go,' and then I just left.

A friend had stayed in Britain and suggested he should try London. So he came, to study and begin a new life.

Adult Intranational Migration

Cultural attitudes concerning the family and sexuality were prominent in the narratives of non-British interviewees who had come to the UK as adults. They were also significant to members of ethnic minorities who had been born and raised here. Thus, a young Asian man had moved to London from the Midlands to study and to live an openly gay lifestyle:

Some friends know I'm gay back home but in London everybody knows. I thought to myself that I can be who I want to be in London, I can start afresh. It's a lot harder to come out back home when, I don't know how to describe it but, with Asian families, it's a lot more difficult. They wouldn't understand, they just wouldn't know what gay means, so that's the reason I never came out to them, but it's a lot better here.

As with the Brazilian respondent above, distance from family had become important for him when, on reaching his mid-twenties, pressures to marry came from his parents. In studying for a degree, he had a reason to leave home, and London beckoned as the centre of gay life in Britain.

Interviewees born in the UK moved to London for a diversity of reasons, but tended to stay in London for factors linked to their sexuality. One man moved into London from the suburbs on meeting a boyfriend. He stayed on in inner London because of the easier availability of gay social networks and 'gay culture':

I started another sort of life. Met my boyfriend and basically started living with him in various places. I had a very gentle sort of coming out.

Another man had moved to London from rural England, originally to study. Again, his integration into gay London life came through a partner:

I come from . . . in the West Country and I moved here when I was a student and stayed on. I lived in student accommodation, then moved in with a partner. I came out in London and went straight into a relationship.

These people had feelings of attachment to their home communities, but they contrasted life in London with the difficulties of being openly gay in small towns or rural communities. Yet another interviewee, who had grown up in a seaside town had this to say:

A   My parents moved down to the coast when I was about two years old. Which is like a very small tiny community, everyone knows everyone else and everyone else's business. And then five years ago I was offered a job in south London. Took the job and been up here ever since.
Q   What was it like living in . . .?
A   It was strange. Looking back now I can see all the faults with it. And although yes it was my home for so many years, I could not live there again. It's just too small and cliquey.

For respondents such as this, the difficulties of living a gay life were not so marked as for interviewees from outside the UK, but the metropolitan pull was strong. As with other examples, though, initial reasons for coming to London were not solely sexual.

Experience of the city is important in the development of socialized gay sexuality (Bech, 1997, Weston, 1995), and gay identities grow in the city into something much greater than a sexual orientation. Migration may be a nodal point in these developments, but we cannot expect it in and of itself to be simply related to sexual desires. This raises an important methodological point. Interviews which ask respondents to provide retrospective accounts of the socialization of their sexualities are almost certain to generate artefacts if they assume any straightforward causality between sexual orientation, migration and area of subsequent residence. Migration may have occurred for no strong reason at the time, but after the development of a strong sexual identity in London, coming to the city may be constructed by the individual, in the light of subsequent events, as being connected with sexuality (in the sense of destiny). A further confounding factor will be relative time spans being studied, which necessarily link with age and stage in the life cycle. Age at migration, and historical changes in attitudes to sexuality in communities of origin, clearly influenced interviewees' narratives.

Age and Migration

Despite what has been said, age and migration may be linked, albeit in complex and changing ways, as data from the following respondents shows. Two interviewees were from the Republic of Ireland. Both had perceived London as providing an easier environment in which to live a gay lifestyle, and one made extensive reference to the restrictions he had previously felt imposed on him by Roman Catholicism. He had come out in Ireland, but had experienced this as difficult, both in terms of family reactions and the fact that the local scene was small and claustrophobic, this being so even for someone from Dublin. The other interviewee was 19 when he came to London, and at the time was not sure of his sexual orientation. To begin with, he classed himself as bisexual and had sex with both men and women. He still (at time of interview) had occasional sex with women but identified as gay, met his female partners at gay clubs, and told all his female partners that he was gay.

The younger age of this last interviewee may be significant, and points to the need to consider changing historical circumstances. We cannot predict how the realization of his sexuality may have differed had he remained in Dublin, but the other Irishman had left Ireland before the decriminalization of homosexuality there, and both spoke of how being gay in Ireland had recently become considerably easier (they made occasional trips home).

This theme was echoed by the Brazilian. Though he spoke in quite negative terms about the possibilities of being gay at home from his own experience, he reported that metropolitan gay life there had considerably improved since he emigrated. In both Brazil and Ireland these perceived changes have occurred in the past five years:

> No the thing is, in Brazil, when I was living in Brazil the gay life used to be difficult, now it's much easier, better than in London they say.

Age bears a complex relation with reasons for migration to London. The age at which an individual recognizes same-sex desires may well not coincide with decisions about lifestyle, identity and social attachment. Even for those men who arrived in London knowing its reputation as a European gay centre, there were usually a number of other attractions, connected with educational, cultural and employment opportunities. London would seem to exert a much more general pull connected with its status and reputation as a world city. Beyond these 'pull' factors, we were struck by the casualness with which some men arrived in London, intending maybe only a short visit or holiday, and then staying on. One Irish interviewee had come to London merely for a holiday, liked it, started working with an uncle who was already in London, and has stayed ever since. It is likely that many more gay men (and very many other people) come for this reason, and find that having someone they already know in the city a useful stepping stone in such a vast and potentially alienating environment.

Residence

The questionnaire survey, in common with other studies, found that there are residential concentrations of gay men within inner London (Annetts, Eisenstadt and Gatter, 1996; Johnson *et al.*, 1994; Kelley, Pebody and Scott, 1996). We also found that gay men tended to be more concentrated in certain boroughs and even postcode areas than others. Thus the borough of Lambeth is more popular than the borough of Lewisham, and within Lambeth, the Brixton area is more popular than other postcodes. This 'clustering' requires explanation. Our interviews provided some insight into this and also helped us to form a picture of how these 'clusters' are experienced by gay men themselves.

It has sometimes been claimed that gay men show little allegiance to their district of residence, tending to be highly mobile around London, moving frequently and not staying within the confines of any one district (Kelley, Pebody and Scott, 1996). While we would agree that gay men seem to show little residential allegiance to particular health authority districts, there does seem to be a pattern of residential concentration once someone has arrived in London within a relatively small number of inner London health authority districts and, more meaningfully, for the men themselves, within certain local-ities. This included, for our interviewees, places seen as 'gay areas' such as Brixton. There was a perception among our informants that many of the areas of inner south London that they lived in were 'quite gay'. This was usually expressed in terms of knowing gay people who lived locally or seeing gay people in the area, such as in the streets. Some spoke of how they felt comfort-able seeing other gay men around or feeling that the area was safe to be visibly gay in. This liking of locale went beyond gay identification: many liked their own area, or south London in general, for a variety of features including parks, restaurants, markets, ethnic diversity, transport links, its cheapness, and the Ritzy Cinema in Brixton.

Brixton was described as having a uniquely attractive ambience. Some felt that it had a specific gay character to it, described by one as being 'working class', that differed from some other 'gay' areas of London, such as Islington or Soho, which were described as being 'pretentious' or 'yuppiefied'. Brixton was clearly well liked for its various facilities and 'cosmopolitan' atmosphere. The diversity of areas, often specifically in terms of ethnicity, is an aspect that has elsewhere been reported as being positively evaluated among gay men (Taylor, Evans and Fraser, 1996). It seems to imply a degree of mutual tolerance, or maybe simply the lack of overall social control by any one group, that gives gay men a social space to inhabit. While the apparent anonymity of the city has been seen as an important factor attracting gay men to large urban centres, it may be that ethnic and other forms of social diversity also play a role.

Choices over where to live were influenced by factors other than liking an area. Often interviewees had moved in to a friend's or boyfriend's place, or found a gay flat share or housing co-op. The emphasis was therefore more on the residence itself than on the area *per se*. It thus becomes hard to disentangle the factors that lead to an area becoming seen as a gay area and which aspects of such an area render it attractive to gay men.

There was a distinction to be made between what attracted gay men to an area initially, often described in terms of chance related to accommodation opportunities, and what made them want to stay in it, described often in terms of positive choice. This distinction reflects what we have already said about migration.

Q Why have you lived where you've lived in London?
A No particular reason. Except where my boyfriend lived. And even if I moved out, I'd live in Brixton because everything's in Brixton and it's not far: the shops, the tube station, railway station, shops, two clubs and one bar, and it's so gay anyways. So, I'd stay in Brixton, I wouldn't go far. Everything's close, close by. So I don't think I'll move, or leave Brixton anyway.

Beyond neighbourhood, particular living spaces were described as 'gay'. This included a local authority housing estate with a large gay population, individual blocks of flats with many gay residents and a lesbian and gay housing cooperative described as 'really close-knit', where residents socialized together, sometimes in the communal garden. Some interviewees lived in gay house or flat shares, with gay flatmates, friends, partners and ex-partners.

There was mention, however, of some tension with what were seen as the local non-gay population, for instance on the Pepys Estate in Deptford (Lewisham) and in Brixton. What are seen as 'gay' or 'gay friendly' areas are not seen as being only that but are also recognized as having other populations and qualities. Areas, especially in cosmopolitan places like inner London, have multiple identities and consequently diverse social meanings for the inhabitants.

Networks and Socializing

Bars are a central institution in gay life (Achilles, 1967; Herdt, 1992). Our survey found, like others (Davies *et al.*, 1993), that bars and clubs are by far the most frequent sites for gay men to meet sexual partners (Annetts, Eisenstadt and Gatter, 1996). We identified three main types of bars and clubs. These were central London venues that attracted clients from a wide geographic area, local venues outside central London that attracted a mainly local clientele and specialist venues that were primarily defined by appeal to a specific population defined by certain characteristics or interests, related to ethnicity, dress code, music and sexual culture, for example. These attract clients from a wide area.

Central London, containing a large number of venues in close proximity, attracted to its bars and clubs nearly all men participating in the questionnaire survey at least occasionally, and nearly half visited them at least weekly. Interviews confirmed this, with many respondents speaking of the convenience of the West End/Soho as a centrally located meeting place for friends who might live in different parts of the city. Particularly for those who worked in central London, its venues are convenient for an after-work drink with work colleagues or other friends. For those travelling across London, the centre of the city provides a convenient stopping-off place as they return home from work or on the way home after a night out.

Some expressed a dislike for the West End bars, preferring the convenience and atmosphere of more local venues in south London. For instance, one interviewee described why he rarely went to the gay bars in the West End:

> I'm quite lazy, I guess. The thought of having to travel home puts me off. And when I do it, about once every three months, it's quite exciting and I have a good time. And I just suppose the places I prefer around where I live, like the Two Brewers (a south London gay pub) is another place that I go to, that I like better as well. But it is just usually the atmosphere of the places. I find them intimidating. Well, I can find them intimidating. Just quite narcissistic. Pretentious.

Not all central London venues are identical, of course, and interviewees had various views on which ones they preferred and why. While some adopted a pub crawl approach, others were loyal to certain bars and were careful to delineate the places they favoured and to explain what distinguished them from those they disliked. But what one disliked another favoured:

> Well I like Kudos [a central London gay bar/cafe] because it's very young and the people who go there, most of them are young. And the music they play there. I like the music. It's modern music and it's really good. That is one of the main reasons I go there, because of the music. And it is very modern, the building.

While it is possible to define the central London venue in terms of location and widespread client catchment area, it is important to recognize the distinctions and meanings that gay men attach to them, whether as an imagined type, the West End or Soho bar, or in terms of the atmosphere and attributes of individual bars.

Local venues were also described primarily in terms of convenience and atmosphere/clientele. Unsurprisingly, to those familiar with going out in London, both the cost and ease of getting to a venue were key issues to many interviewees. Local places were thus attractive, particularly to those without access to a car and those on more limited budgets. While many informants tended to socialize mainly in south London, given the amount of gay venues in the area, proximity (26 venues in the three boroughs constituting LSL) was not seen as the only or even main consideration in choice of venue. The atmosphere of a place, for instance, plays an important part.

Specialist venues, which tend to be clubs rather than bars, cover a broad range of 'interest groups'. This includes drugs (such as Ecstasy) and dance clubs, leather and SM venues, uniform nights, 'bears' nights, backroom sex clubs, nights aimed at certain racial and ethnic groups such as Black or Southeast Asian gay men. Interviewees were generally willing to leave south London, if need be, to attend these places. They were often their favourite venues and seemed to attract a degree of loyalty.

Some were key sites for men who saw themselves as part of a certain 'scene' or social network, while others were spoken of more in terms of a specific 'night' or 'event', although these overlapped. It is therefore misleading to focus purely on specific venues. Specialist nights and the key sites of certain networks may change venue location, taking their clientele with them or only inhabit a venue on a certain night of the week or month. For instance, one man spoke of being 'into' uniforms and therefore travelled around London to any uniform nights. Another man described how his favourite club night was Bulk, a club for large men, that had initially been 'in tottering' distance from his home in south London, but which he now visited at the venue in west London it had relocated to. In this way a certain venue may be a local venue on some nights and several different specialist venues on other nights. Therefore, while some venues have a defined status as a specialist venue, e.g. a dance/drugs venue, it would be wrong to focus solely on venues and not on the scenes they house.

Choices of Gay Venue

A key factor in the choice of venue for an individual is the desired purpose of the visit. Meeting friends for a drink, going out for a 'fun' night of dancing and drugs with a regular crowd of clubbing friends or seeking easily available sexual partners, may dictate a quite different choice of venue. Although many interviewees had quite defined and regular patterns of venue use, this did not mean they were regulars at only one type of venue. Depending on the people accompanying, if any, and depending on the intended purpose of the visit, very different types of venue could be selected by the same person:

Q   Why do you like Duckie [a weekly night at a local venue] so much?
A   I like it because it's the opposite of going to Substation South [a local venue]. Substation South is sort of like a sexually charged atmosphere, which I like, but if I just want to go out and have fun with my friends, I go to a place like Duckie because it is a mixture of men and women and it is really relaxed, really crowded and you just get drunk and dance and be silly.

Some of the men we spoke to described how their attitude towards a venue was influenced by their attitude towards the 'type' of gay men to be found there. Type could be related to a variety of factors, including age, ethnicity, drug use, physical appearance and a distinction between 'hard' and 'fluffy' or 'queeny'.

> I won't go anywhere that is completely fluffy and non-drug-taking and non-shagging like GAY, that is full of 19, 20-year-olds. Like people who think that a sniff of poppers and you become a heroin addict, and like wanting to get to know somebody before they sleep with you.

Concern was expressed not only with the 'types' of gay men respondents tended to be sexually interested in, but also in the general atmosphere of the place:

> Since they let women in there now, I hate the place. Not because it's women, it's because the crowd has tended to change as well. It used to be a fairly heavy crowd that was going there, but now you are getting too many prissy queens. I do not like prissy queens. I can put up with them and talk to them, but I don't really want to socialize with them.

Some men felt excluded from venues because they did not fit the 'type' that went there:

> I mean Heaven [a gay venue] always was to me a slag ground, you know, it's where you shag people. It's, it's you've got to be trendy. If you're not young, if you're not pretty, then you might as well not be there.

Other key factors in choice of venue that were apparent from our interviews included financial outlay, the type of music played, and the consumption (or not) of alcohol and drugs. The frequency of visiting gay venues varied considerably in both the questionnaire survey and interviews, with some men going out almost every night while others did so rarely.

Friendship Networks

Respondents were asked about their networks of friends – who they were and how they socialized with them. Some of the men had virtually exclusively gay friends; while other interviewees reported a mixture of friends of diverse sexuality, whom they associated with differently according to context. As might be expected, straight men tended to be a minority in the friendship networks of gay men, outside the context of the workplace:

> I've got a few lesbian friends ... and I have heterosexual women friends as well. I don't think I actually know any straight men. When I think about it, I don't really mix with heterosexual men at all, apart if they are sort of through family or through work or something, but I can honestly say I don't have any heterosexual male friends.

Another man commented on the quality of the friendships he had with straight men at work

> We have a sort of hearty relationship and go out to straight pubs or visit each other's houses.

The degree of exclusivity in how gay an individual's friendship networks were did, however, vary:

> There are the people I go drinking with that I work with, and then some of those carry over to people I go out to town with. And one of them, one girl that carries over, that goes out clubbing and every-thing. A significant number of them are straight men, and it is getting less gay men, more straight men. Still not so many lesbians.

Several respondents had close relationships with straight women friends, pro-viding mutual support over emotional issues. One man distinguished discuss-ing emotions with women friends and sex with gay male friends:

> With straight people [women] it's usually more the subject is affairs of the heart, whereas with gay people it's what went down.

There were varying degrees of overlap between social circles. Compart-mentalizing was one strategy employed by some to control knowledge of their sexual identity. One man had mainly gay friends, but also played for a local sports club, in which he was not 'out'. For reasons of confidentiality he kept his socializing with the sports club completely separate from the rest of his social life. Compartmentalizing was also a strategy used in organizing other aspects of socializing. Some men, for example, sometimes took women friends to gay venues because they reported that the women enjoyed the atmosphere and felt relatively safe from predatory straight men. At other times they took specific gay male friends with them when they went out to find sexual partners. Taking straight male friends to gay venues could, however, be more problematic. One man discussing his straight flatmates said:

> I don't really want to socialize with them. They've got their own friends and if I want to go out I want to go to a gay club. They wouldn't mind going but I'm sure they wouldn't like it. I know that because they are really good looking, they'd get their arse pinched and stuff like that. I don't want gay people to get a bad name by taking them, and them getting touched up and stuff, and then telling their friends.

Compartmentalization has been described by sociologists as a feature of life for people who, to use Goffman's term, have some stigma (in this case, minority sexuality) which makes them discreditable to the majority (Goffman, 1963). Elsewhere it has been discussed in relation to gay men with particular reference to the process of 'information management' in relation to coming out (Davies, 1992).

Disability, Ethnicity and Gay Community

Social networks were also shaped by other factors such as disability and ethnicity. Two interviewees were deaf, and both men highlighted the ways in which this affected their participation within gay community. One was excited by his first experience of the gay scene, but frustrated by communication problems:

> Because I was a new face, everybody looked at me and picked me up. Yeah. Everyone was very friendly. There was just one problem and that was communication.

These men described social networks of deaf gay men that formed a community within the gay community which provided opportunities for social interaction and mutual support:

> I go to Brothers and Sisters club [for deaf lesbians and gay men] so I can relax and be signing with everyone, which makes communication easy. I don't go there for sex and relationships.

Disability is thus a focus of social organization and social exclusion within the gay community, as it is within wider society, although this may be changing:

> But more and more the attitude is changing within the gay community. The hearing gay are now really supporting the deaf gay through local councils and in the gay community. It's really improving. Interpreters, more interpreters now. The Lighthouse [a centre providing services to people with HIV and AIDS] in London, they welcome the deaf.

Gay men from various ethnic groups in London have formed many different social networks organized around ethnicity. In this study we identified many such networks, sometimes organized around specific nights at gay venues or informal parties. These included networks for Southeast Asian, South Asian, Turkish, Cypriot, Latin American, including Colombian and Brazilian, and African/Caribbean gay and bisexual men (Annetts, Eisenstadt and Gatter, 1996). They cater both for men who have migrated to the UK and for those born into ethnic minority communities within the UK. These spaces and networks can provide support to new migrants and safe spaces against racism in the gay community.

These scenes within the gay scene are sometimes based in commercial venues, on certain nights of the week or month, but they are also organized around more informal or temporary spaces. This may be partly a reflection of a relative lack of economic power of ethnic minority gay men. One man described such a Black gay scene:

> But I mean there are, you know, it's people's homes, the occasional paying party, you know what I mean, that people have a blues. You know, it's just finding the space and taking it over for a night and having a party there. . . . What's been happening over the past four to five years is that there are certain bodies of people that have come together as a collective and organized parties over, say, four to five months, once a month, and those last for a while.

Experiences of racism, sexual objectification and cultural difference can lead to the exclusion of ethnic minority gay men from the spaces of the 'mainstream' scene and the development of separate gay networks organized around 'race' and ethnicity. For instance, one man preferred using an HIV service centre on a designated night for Black service users rather than the gay designated night:

> I don't like it because, even with gay night, when you go in there you kind of feel left out, because not a lot of Black gay men go there. You're just going to feel out of place, so I don't really go there. And

most of the time when you go there, people, all they ever do is eye you up. When you go there the only thing they are interested in is your body, that is all they want.

Another Black interviewee discussed his experiences in terms of being involved in friendship networks and organizations for Black lesbians and gay men, as well as 'mainstream' gay culture:

So my friends are quite mixed but I don't tend to mix them together because actually there has been quite a clash and stuff. I see them in different settings, different venues. My Black friends tend to be mainly in Black clubs or Black focus bars or maybe some sort of workshops around some sort of Black gay issues and in my home or their home. I would say probably for my white friends it would be mainly sort of the mainstream bars which would be The Edge or Kudos or something like that.

Conclusions

On the basis of this exploratory investigation, we cannot make any strong theoretical claims. There are, however, certain prominent emergent themes which are relevant to theorizing gay community participation and practical suggestions for HIV prevention, treatment and care.

Our broad orientation has been social constructionism mixed with symbolic interactionism: we have chosen to see community and identity as being located symbolically as well as spatially, and see both community and identity meaning what their inhabitants make them mean. Epstein (1987) has argued, however, that people are not totally free to construct identities and communities just as they please. Instead, there are certain material, structural and discursive constraints which create the outer limits to social creativity. In agreement with part of his argument, we found that choices over residence and socializing are circumscribed by material considerations.

We have also seen how disability and ethnicity plays a complex role in relation to processes of inclusion and exclusion. Unacceptable sexuality can lead to exclusion from or self-distancing from family or community of origin. Thus, sexuality played a notable role in narratives of migration. On the other hand, ethnicity can lead to exclusion *within* adopted gay communities. Identity factors such as race, ethnicity and disability cross-cut sexual identity and shape the experience of being gay. This is to suggest that multiple belongings problematize totalizing conceptions of identity and community (Deverell and Prout, 1995).

In discussing residence we saw how places such as Brixton become 'imagined' gay communities (Anderson, 1991). The visible presence of gay men can lead to a sense of ownership of space, though there is always awareness that other communities are present, with whom there may be common cause or tension. Territory is both actual and symbolic. Areas of cities may become symbolized as gay because gay men come to have a sense of safety there, even if in empirical terms they are in a minority (Myslik, 1996).

Our data also illustrates diversity within gay community at a level below major social divisions such as ethnicity. There are, on the one hand, specialist social networks based on sexual and recreational tastes. On the other hand, there are different social networks between which a single individual may move, which are located in different social spaces (such as the club for sex versus the club for dancing with women friends). These networks may be exclusive (as when a not fully out gay man compartmentalizes his life) or they may have varying degrees of overlap in time and space. The complexity of social networks and the degrees to which they intersect or are held separate by their participants are highly relevant to new thinking about HIV prevention.

Elsewhere we have suggested that the migration of large numbers of gay men to London and their concentration, both residentially and in terms of gay venues, within inner London, suggests a commensurate targeting of resources (Annetts, Eisenstadt and Gatter, 1996). It may also be important to consider what effects this ongoing migrancy on the London gay population might be, perhaps in terms of support networks, community-based strategies and diversity in terms of language, national origin and ethnicity. New arrivals may need targeting to facilitate an understanding of, and access to, services.

The residential concentration of gay men has implications for locality-based services in inner London. This is most important in those areas where the greatest numbers of gay men reside. While London's gay male population seems to be highly mobile in terms of both residence and patterns of venue usage, it is important to recognize that this is largely within and across a small number of health authorities (Annetts, Eisenstadt and Gatter, 1996; Kelley, Pebody and Scott, 1996; Johnson *et al.*, 1994).

Mobility is not the same for all gay men. While many men use the gay scene venues of central London regularly, others do not; they have social lives that are more local or based in more informal and private spaces. Regularity and intensity of gay scene participation is also varied and changes over time. Consequently, sexual health promotion strategies that focus only on gay scene commercial venues will miss many men. Scene-focused strategies need to take into account the multiple functions that gay venues serve and the diversity of venue types, their clientele, and the social networks of clientele which extend beyond the individual venues.

It is important to contextualize often crude questionnaire data concerning the social lives of gay men in terms of the multiple, changing and diverse networks in which they participate. Notions of 'the gay community' and 'the gay scene', or even more specific ones such as 'Black gay men' or 'the gay bar', may be too restricted in the way they are currently deployed in relation to service provision. We urge caution in making assumptions about the relationship between the population incidence of homosexuality, or even gay identity, and participation in the gay community and 'the scene'. Focusing on the participation of individuals in multiple, diverse and changing social networks potentially provides a more realistic description of the social lives of gay men whatever their age, ethnicity or other identifying factors. These networks may be localized or London-wide, may include people who are not gay men, and may overlap. They are also shaped by those factors of social stratification and exclusion that shape wider society, such as age, 'race', wealth, disability, and so on. Gay men are members of many different social networks, including many that are not based on shared sexual identity. Commissioning and provision of services need to take these networks into account, recognizing that the lives of gay men cannot be described using simplistic categories but need to be seen in their full complexity and diversity.

Acknowledgement

The research described in this paper was funded by Lambeth, Southwark and Lewisham Health Authority and was conducted jointly between South Bank University and the HIV Project. Jason Annetts and Kevin Eisenstadt were the researchers, managed by Katie Deverell (HIV Project) and Philip Gatter (South Bank University), respectively. Katie Deverell and Philip Gatter authored the research proposal, and the project was managed overall by James Barratt, Director of the HIV Project, and Professor Jeffrey Weeks (South Bank University).

Notes

1 They used a mixture of unstructured individual interviews, group interviews, focus groups, participant observation and textual analysis.
2 In one sense all sexuality must be socialized, and psychoanalysis would take this view. We use this phrase more sociologically to refer to the process of developing a sexuality in the individual's changing social circumstances.
3 Care must be taken in comparing the results of the two studies, since different questions were asked. It is not clear how the question 'Where did you grow up?' was interpreted in the GMFA study. The question of place of birth is different.
4 Again, care must be taken in comparing different studies. There are methodological problems in comparing questions about sexual behaviours with those focused on social identities (Annetts, 1996).
5 The 15 men interviewed ranged in age from 21 to 35 years; mean age and median age were both 28 years. The men represented a wide range of ethnicities: White UK, White Irish, White Australian, White New Zealander, Black UK, Black Caribbean, Black Asian, Latin American and

Black African. The elapsed time spent in London ranged from less than one year to an entire lifetime (32 years). Most had migrated to London from elsewhere in the UK or elsewhere in the world. Four were born in London, two of whom left as children and returned in adulthood. Two of our interviewees were deaf.

References

ACHILLES, N. (1967) 'The development of the homosexual bar as an institution', in Gagnon, J. and Simon, W. (eds) *Sexual Deviance*. New York: Harper & Row.

ALTMAN, D. (1986) *AIDS and the New Puritanism*. London: Pluto Press.

ALTMAN, D. (1994) *Power and Community: Organizational and Cultural Responses to AIDS*. London: Taylor & Francis.

ALTMAN, D. (1997) 'The global gay: discursive and institutional prerequisites'. Paper given at Beyond Boundaries: Sexuality Across Culture, First International Conference, Amsterdam, 29 July to 1 August 1997.

ANDERSON, B. (1991) *Imagined Communities: Reflections on the Origin and Spread of Nationalism*. London: Verso.

ANNETTS, J. (1996) *Mapping (homo)sexuality: a critical review of the literature on the incidence and distribution of male homosexuality*. Working Paper 1, Lambeth, Southwark and Lewisham's Gay and Bisexual Men's HIV and AIDS Prevention Services Review and Social Mapping Project. London: HIV Project.

ANNETTS, J., EISENSTADT, K. and GATTER, P. (1996) *Gay and Bisexual Men's HIV Prevention Service Review and Social Mapping Project: Final Report*. London: Lambeth, Southwark and Lewisham Health Authority.

BAO, J. (1997) 'Transnational migration and sexual identity'. Paper given at Beyond Boundaries: Sexuality Across Culture, First International Conference, Amsterdam, 29 July to 1 August 1997.

BECH, H. (1997) *When Men Meet: Homosexuality and Modernity*. Cambridge: Polity Press.

BELL, D. and VALENTINE, G. (eds) (1995) *Mapping Desire: Geographies of Sexualities*. London: Routledge.

BRIGHTON OURSTORY PROJECT (1992) *Daring Hearts: Lesbian and Gay Lives of 50s and 60s Brighton*. Brighton: Queens Park Books.

CANT, B. (ed.) (1997) *Invented Moralities? Lesbians and Gays Talk about Migration*. London: Cassell.

CARRILO, H. (1997) 'Hybrid sexual cultures in modern Mexico: implications for the practice of AIDS prevention'. Paper given at Beyond Boundaries: Sexuality Across Culture, First International Conference, Amsterdam, 29 July to 1 August 1997.

CASTELLS, M. (1983) *The City and the Grassroots*. Berkeley, CA: University of California Press.

Coxon, A. (1985) *The 'Gay Lifestyle' and the Impact of AIDS*. Project SIGMA Working Paper 1. London: Project SIGMA.

Davies, P. (1992) 'The role of disclosure in coming out among gay men', in Plummer, K. (ed.) *Modern Homosexualities: Fragments of Lesbian and Gay Experience*. London: Routledge.

Davies, P., Hickson, F., Hunt, A. and Weatherburn, P. (1993) *Sex, Gay Men and AIDS*. London: Taylor & Francis.

Deverell, K. and Prout, A. (1995) 'Sexuality, identity and community – reflections on the MESMAC project', in Aggleton, P., Davies, P. and Hart, G. (eds) *AIDS: Safety, Sexuality and Risk*. London: Taylor & Francis.

Dowsett, G. and McInnes, D. (1996) '"Post-AIDS": assessing the long-term social impact of HIV/AIDS in gay communities'. Oral presentation to the XIth International Conference on AIDS, Vancouver, Canada, 7–12 July 1996.

Dowsett, G. *et al.* (1992) 'Gay men, HIV/AIDS and social research: an Antipodean perpective', in Aggleton, P., Davies, P. and Hart, G. (eds) *AIDS: Rights, Risk and Reason*. London: Falmer Press.

Epstein, S. (1987) 'Gay politics, ethnic identity: the limits of social constructionism', *Socialist Review* **93/94**, pp. 9–54.

Gatter, P. (1995) 'Anthropology, HIV and contingent identities', *Social Science and Medicine* **41**, 11, pp. 1523–33.

Goffman, E. (1963) *Stigma: Notes on the Management of Spoiled Identity*. Englewood Cliffs, NJ: Prentice Hall.

Hart, G. and Boulton, M. (1995) 'Sexual behaviour in gay men: towards a sociology of risk', in Aggleton, P., Davies, P. and Hart, G. (Eds) *AIDS: Safety, Sexuality and Risk*. London: Taylor & Francis.

Herdt, G. (ed.) (1992) *Gay Culture in America: Essays from the Field*. Boston, MA: Beacon Press.

Johnson, A., Wellings, K., Wadsworth, J. and Field, J. (1994) *Sexual Attitudes and Lifestyles*. Oxford: Blackwell Scientific.

Kelley, P., Pebody, R. and Scott, P. (1996) *How Far Will You Go? A Survey of London Gay Men's Migration and Mobility*. London: Gay Men Fighting AIDS.

Kippax, S., Connell, R., Dowsett, G. and Crawford, J. (1993) *Sustaining Safe Sex: Gay Communities Respond to AIDS*. London: Taylor & Francis.

Levine, M. (1979) 'Gay ghetto', in Levine, M. (ed.) *Gay Men: The Sociology of Male Homosexuality*. New York: Harper & Row.

Michael, R. *et al.* (1994) *Sex in America: A Definitive Survey*. London: Little, Brown & Co.

Mort, F. (1996) *Cultures of Consumption: Masculinities and Social Space in Late Twentieth Century Britain*. London: Routledge.

Myslik, W.D. (1996) 'Renegotiating the social/sexual identities of place', in Duncan, N. (ed.) *Body Space*. London: Routledge.

Nardi, P. and Schneider, B. (1998) *Social Perspectives in Lesbian and Gay Studies: A Reader.* London: Routledge.

Plummer, K. (1998) 'Afterword: the past, present and futures of the sociology of same-sex relations', in Nardi, P. and Schneider, B. (eds) *Social Perspectives in Lesbian and Gay Studies: A Reader.* London: Routledge.

Tan, M. (1995) 'From *Bakla* to gay: shifting gender identities and sexual behaviours in the Philippines', in Parker, R. and Gagnon, J. (eds) *Conceiving Sexuality: Approaches to Sex Research in a Postmodern World.* London: Routledge.

Taylor, I., Evans, K. and Fraser, P. (1996) *A Tale of Two Cities: Global Change, Local Feeling and Everyday Life in the North of England. A Study in Manchester and Sheffield.* London: Routledge.

Watney, S. (1993) 'Emergent sexual identities and HIV/AIDS', in Aggleton, P., Davies, P. and Hart, G. (eds) *AIDS: Facing the Second Decade.* London: Falmer Press.

Weston, K. (1995) 'Get thee to a big city: sexual imaginary and the great gay migration', *GLQ* **2/3**, pp. 253–77.

Chapter 8

Observing the Rules: An Ethnographic Study of London's Cottages and Cruising Areas

Peter Keogh and Paul Holland

Research into public sex environments (PSEs) falls into two phases, the first beginning in the late 1960s and the second at the start of the AIDS epidemic in the mid-1980s. Of the earlier phase, the best-known study is Humphreys' *Tearoom Trade* (1970), which marks a burgeoning literature on this topic (Bell and Weinberg, 1978; Styles, 1979; Delph, 1978; Ponte, 1974). Such studies concentrated on the 'type of men frequenting PSEs and contributed to a dominant conception of these venues as used mainly by heterosexually identified, covert homosexuals in order to avoid stigma while achieving sexual pleasure. This conception re-emerged early in the HIV epidemic when PSEs were characterized as sites where HIV might be transmitted from the gay population to the heterosexual population. Moreover, it was often assumed that men frequenting PSEs would not be part of a gay community and would therefore not be 'reached' by interventions targeting gay men. However, PSEs are not the exclusive domain of behaviourally bisexual heterosexually identified men. A recent study of gay men in the UK (Keogh *et al.*, 1998), shows that 30 per cent had met a partner in a cruising area and 20 per cent had met a partner in a cottage in the previous year. Likewise, Weatherburn *et al.* (1996) show that PSEs are merely one of a range of places used by behaviourally bisexual men to access same-sex partners.

In the UK, PSEs are generally of two types. Public toilets (known as cottages) are often used by men to engage in anonymous sexual encounters. Parks, heaths and scrublands (cruising areas) are also used, as are motorway stopovers, beaches, and so on. Such sites are generally well known to local men seeking anonymous sex and will function as PSEs sometimes for a few months (perhaps during the summer) but more frequently, will have lives spanning decades or even hundreds of years. There are few studies which seek to establish why certain public spaces facilitate sexual interaction whereas others do not. Such a question is of more than academic interest. HIV prevention outreach has been carried out in PSEs in the UK as far back as 1988 (Aggleton *et al.*, 1992) yet it remains to be established whether outreach is the best intervention and if not, what might be more appropriate. Moreover, if any risk reduction intervention is to be successful, it is necessary to identify the factors which influence the sexual and social behaviour of men participating in sex on the sites. Although something is known about the erotic and practical motivations of men frequenting PSEs (Church *et al.*, 1993; Keogh *et al.*, 1993), little is known about the role of the site itself in facilitating sexual risk taking. Knowledge of such factors may enable us to make a systematic assessment of a PSE in order to determine what is the likely sexual risk behaviour there and what, if any, interventions are appropriate.

Such a study requires an analysis of the physical nature and social uses of the space as well as detailed observation of the interactions of men using it. Delph (1978) describes such interactions as a series of stages, in which individuals use silent cues and reciprocal actions to signal their mutual intentions and their sexual interest in each other. Thus, participants manipulate physical and social variables in order to bring about sexual ends. This chapter is a microanalysis of cruising and cottaging behaviour which identifies how such physical and social variables are manipulated and how they interact with certain types of behaviour in order to bring about sexual ends. We examine sites which display variation across a range of variables in order to identify features (both physical and social) which were common to all sites and behaviours. We researched sexual and social interaction at four very different PSEs. We first look at the features common to all of them and then explore the nature of the relationship between these features and sexual or social behaviour on the sites, highlighting a number of key themes.

Thirty PSEs in London were visited and observed for a short period of time. An analysis of this data yielded a list of dimensions by which each site was assessed (e.g. whether the site is accessible by foot, by car or by public transport; what the site is normally used for; the amount of temporal or seasonal variation in the levels of sexual activity on the site). Sites with maximum variability along these dimensions were selected and participant observation was carried out at these sites over a twelve-month period.

A reflexive, inductive methodology was used for observation and logging data. Thus, sites were observed in order to record behaviour, and these observations were analysed to provide the conceptual framework with which to interpret behaviour. A chronological narrative account of actions, movements, changes in physical settings and events was made. The quality of the field notes was ensured by recording verbatim accounts as opposed to paraphrasing; by applying critical questioning and designating degrees of reliability to observations; by using concrete descriptive language as much as possible; by raising critical questions for further fieldwork within the notes; and by inserting memos and interpretations into the notes, building upon themes. Notes were made promptly.

Observations were divided into conceptual categories. Early observations on sites, or observations of new phenomena were determined as descriptive observations (Loftland and Loftland, 1995). From these descriptive observations, it was possible to pose questions to be answered in further focused observations. These may or may not in their turn give rise to further descriptive observations from which further questions could be asked. There were two main organizing principles for logging data. The first was to divide the site geographically into zones. The second was to divide these zones according to a range of criteria (e.g. users' behaviour in each zone, the geography of the zone, the meanings that zones hold for users). This demarcation was particularly useful for the larger cruising areas. An analytic-inductive methodology (Znaniecki, 1934; Burgess, 1991) was used to analyse the field notes. In this approach, an instance (or event) is explained in terms of a likely hypothesis. This hypothesis is expanded, modified or abandoned by comparisons with other similar instances and an inclusive description thus attained. The methodology suited the very factual accounts recorded in the field notes. This chapter is based on an analysis of observation notes from four very different sites. The sites were observed for a total of 216 hours over a twelve-month period.

Mill Street Cottage

Mill Street Cottage is a free-standing public toilet located just off a busy high street in southeast London. Inside the space measures approximately 8 m × 4 m with five cubicles facing a wall of urinals. There is a separate washroom approximately 2 m × 3 m in size. The cottage is open from 8.00 am to 5.00 pm and is busy for much of the time with cottagers and others.

Avon Cemetery

Avon Cemetery is located in the northeast part of central London. It is an early Victorian cemetery with one main path running the entire distance of the cemetery, from which many smaller paths deviate. In between are areas of dense bush, ivy and gravestones. There are several benches scattered along the paths. Most of the cruising occurs at the rear of the cemetery, along the main path and the paths running off it. This is a popular area for cruisers and others, especially on warmer days.

The Railway Sidings

The Railway Sidings is an area of dense bushland sandwiched between a railway track and a large public park in north London. It is traversed by one main pathway from its top to its bottom with two smaller paths deviating from this top path. These paths in turn lead to a densely wooded area of bush with smaller trodden paths running through it. The area is separated from the park by a long chain-link fence which is breached in one place. There are entrances to the area at either end of the sidings. The site is sometimes used as a short cut for people going from the nearby train station to the largely residential area behind the park; however, such users will rarely wander into the seemingly impenetrable wooded area. Hence this area is used predominantly by cruisers. Because it is rarely disturbed, almost total overall privacy is assured.

Fern Park

Fern Park is a formal inner-city park in south central London. It is encompassed by three main roads and a smaller access road at the rear. Cruising is concentrated around a shop, seating area and public toilet. The park is busy all year round, especially in summer. Likewise, the shop is open all year round and acts as a congregation area for park users and cruisers. The toilet itself is quite small (approximately $3\,m \times 4\,m$) with three cubicles against one wall and a disabled toilet and wash area on the other. The urinals are actually structurally separate from the main toilet. All the sexual activity on the site occurs within the toilet. This is because the park is very open with a formal arrangement of paths and beds with no real bushland.

The Central Features of PSEs

The most important unifying feature of public sex is its subversive use of public spaces. Since there are no specially designed PSEs (as there are say, shopping centres or factories), public sexual activities make use of pre-existing public spaces which are more or less suited to that purpose. A place is suited to public sex activity when its legitimate patterns of behaviour can be easily subverted. There are two general elements which determine this. These are the nature of the place's social predetermination and the extent of the place's spatial predetermination.

Spatial Predetermination

Spatial predetermination is the extent to which the site is determined by physical objects: boundaries (walls, fences, bushes); internal arrangement (pathways, passages, walls, divisions, screens, etc.); and the proximity of the place to other significant places (such as roads, shops, offices, parks).

Social Predetermination

Nearly all civic public places are built or formed in order to carry out a predetermined function. This function is fulfilled by a finite range of appropriate behaviours. Other behaviours, though possible are not socially appropriate. Thus, for example, it is socially appropriate to walk up and down aisles of a supermarket and stand in a queue, etc. It is, however, not socially appropriate to recline on the counter-tops. Likewise, in a swimming pool, it is not socially appropriate for a man to appear in the women's changing room (or vice versa) or to appear naked in the foyer (although to do so in the men's changing rooms would not excite much interest). The PSEs studied exist in either highly socially and spatially predetermined places (e.g. Mill Street Cottage or Fern Park), or in what we have called 'non-places', that is, places which are not socially predetermined, i.e. they have no social or civic function, but which are spatially predetermined. An example of this type of site is the Railway Sidings; other examples might include ruined buildings or parks and commons at night. The key to understanding the relationship between the social and spatial predetermination of a place and the public sexual activity that occurs there is to understand the extent to which predetermined rules of engagement or interactions (i.e. socially appropriate behaviour) can be subverted in order to facilitate covert sexual activity.

The interaction of spatial and social predetermining factors gives rise to three further conditions, the presence of which will determine whether a site will be used for sex and the nature of sexual interaction at that site. We can call them access, privacy and relations of proximity.

Access

How access is gained to the site and who is allowed on the site are highly constitutive of the nature of sexual activity there. The site may be accessible to men only (e.g. Mill Street Cottage), inaccessible to any but the most determined of interlopers (e.g. the Railway Sidings) or accessible to everyone (e.g. Fern Park or Avon Cemetery).

Privacy

The amount of privacy that the site affords is also important. Sites range from those which provide privacy to the whole person at all times (e.g. the Railway Sidings) to those which may only screen the slightest sexual touch for a matter of seconds (Mill Street Cottage).

Relations of Proximity

How close or how distant men can get to each other is also formative of sexual contact on the site. Thus, some sites allow men to be in such close bodily proximity that sexual contact can be achieved merely through a straying hand. Others, however, allow men to gain sufficient distance for a sufficient amount of time to allow the exchange of meaningful glances, stares and bodily movements.

For example, the social predetermination of Mill Street Cottage is particular in a number of respects. Firstly, it is a male-only space. Secondly, it is socially acceptable to hold one's penis in one's hand while standing in close proximity to another man. This social predetermination interacts with the spatial predetermination to provide further features which makes the site most appropriate to public sexual activity. The internal organization of the cottage affords relationships of proximity which allow men to determine and exhibit their sexual intentions (distinguish themselves from ordinary users), to establish mutual sexual interest and to engage in sexual acts in privacy without getting 'caught'. Therefore, the active cottage is a space where social and spatial predeterminations interact to produce the right type of access, the best relations of proximity and the right type of privacy. In addition, the enactment of sexual encounters is simultaneous to the space's use for its legitimate purpose. Thereby, the two uses of the space never or rarely conflict:

> The first person to come in went straight to the first urinal and did a pee – he was straight. . . . After about ten minutes a guy wearing a suit came in and stood at one of the urinals in the middle. At first I thought that he was straight as he did not really look as he entered and he didn't really 'check the cottage out' then he left without peeing. . . . Eventually a young guy came in and stood at the urinals. He was directly followed by the guy wearing a suit. The young guy was very observant of me and of where the other guy was going. The suited guy went to the third cubicle, then to the end cubicle and then back to the third cubicle, where he eventually closed the door. The young guy looked at me a couple of times and then left. I think he was interested but was not sure about it. The suit guy came out of the cubicle shortly after and then left the cottage. I stayed at the urinal. A couple of minutes later, the suit guy came back into the cottage and stood at the urinal immediately next to me. He then stood back so I could see his penis. (Field notes, Mill Street Cottage)

Similarly, cruising areas in public parks allow for a limited set of socially predetermined actions (sitting, walking aimlessly, standing and staring, etc). However, they are spatially predetermined to ensure certain relations of proximity which in themselves facilitate the game of increasingly sexualized reciprocal gestures. The proximity of a bench to a path allows two men to exchange meaningful glances, the proximity of the path to another path allows one man to lead while another follows, etc., thus allowing two men to indicate that they are mutually sexually interested. The privacy provided by the twists in the paths and the overgrown bushy areas allows these men to achieve sexual contact. Therefore, men can define their identity as cruisers, establish mutual sexual interest and engage in sex all within a space that is simultaneously used by others:

I kept walking when I came across a bearded guy in his late thirties. As I approached him, he looked at me and I looked back. He stopped after a few metres as if to indicate interest. I also stopped and slowly began to follow. When he came to the dissecting path, he took it. He walked down to the end and stopped. I stopped at the other end. Eventually he came down to my end and, as he passed me, he said hello. I said hello to him and stayed where I was. He waked about 25 metres down and stopped, facing me and looking at me for most of the time. (Field notes, Avon Cemetery)

A guy walked by and cruised me (looked at my eyes and my crotch). Then went and stood where the other two had been (roughly 10 yards away). He then walked by again and went on to the other path. I got up and followed him. He had stopped a couple of metres down. I walked past him and sat on a block of cement. He walked by me and stopped to my right, then he started rubbing his penis through his pants. (Field notes, Avon Cemetery)

This analysis becomes more useful when we explore how the specific relationships between social and spatial predeterminations of a site influence the cruising or cottaging that occurs there. All the public sex encounters observed took place in three stages. Defining behaviour allows cruisers or cottagers to distinguish each other from other people. Through certain reciprocal gestures, interested behaviour confirms a mutual sexual interest between two or more men. Finally, there is some form of sexual contact. Each stage was wholly dependent upon the successful completion of the preceding one. Therefore, interest is never declared unless both players have defined themselves as public sex participants. Sex is rarely if ever initiated unless it has been established that there is a mutual sexual interest. In this way, mistakes are seldom made and the wrong man is rarely propositioned.

The types of communication used by men to pass through these stages was generally of two types. In highly scripted interaction, different men use the same actions or sequences of actions repeatedly, almost like choreographed dance (e.g. men who walk past each other, look at each other, stop, turn to look at each other again). On the other hand, individualistic communication depended on interactions arising both from the individual situation and those men involved (activity characterized by verbal utterances, individual gestures, smiles, winks, etc.). This analysis allows us to establish a range of relations between the nature of the site, the types of communication that occur there and the type of sex that is likely to happen (Figure 8.1).

Generally speaking, the more the site is spatially and socially predetermined, the more scripted the types of interaction. For example, sites easily accessed and used by others (e.g. Mill Street Cottage or Fern Park) offer a strictly limited set of acceptable actions by which it is possible to define oneself as a cruiser or cottager, indicate interest and achieve sexual contact. However,

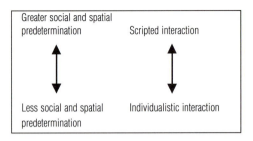

Figure 8.1   Relation between interaction and determination of site.

these limitations are often precisely what facilitates successful sexual contact. There is a simple and limited set of unequivocal actions that could be interpreted in one of two ways.

There is a simple binary opposition in Mill Street Cottage, for example. A man entering either glances or he does not. He either goes to a certain urinal or he does not. He either urinates or he does not, he either looks or he does not. Likewise, when cruising in Fern Park a man either looks or he does not, he either walks purposively or he does not, he either stops or he does not. When taken all together, these actions constitute a simple language of either positive or negative signals. This binary reciprocal interpretive language communicates complex desires in the absence of verbal or gestural signals.

In the case of less socially and spatially predetermined sites, behaviours are generally of the latter individualistic type. Those sites that are hardly socially or spatially predetermined at all (e.g. the Railway Sidings) offer a particular configuration of the three elements of privacy, relations of proximity and access. Rarely frequented by others, they offer unlimited access to public sex participants. Because of this, they provide a 'cover' of privacy. This may be a literal cover of impenetrable bush, or may be the cover of darkness in parkland at night. There is therefore no established set of socially predetermined rituals that are common or acceptable to this environment, no 'innocent' behaviours which cover subversive ones. Instead, social organization is determined entirely by the primary function of the site (i.e. the sexual function).

In these sites it is unmediated sexual imperatives that shape behaviour. Therefore, cruisers will walk around the site, not because the way they walk could be interpreted as significant, but because walking in a certain direction or route ensures that one can see as many men on the site as possible in the shortest possible time. In a similar manner, the interaction between the cruisers is not coded, but direct and individualistic. Men will smile, wink and make overt sexual passes at each other without having gone through an earlier codified defining process. The imperative to define intentions becomes less important as the site will generally only contain men who are there for sex, exhibiting their intention in a direct (as opposed to coded) manner:

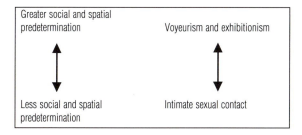

Figure 8.2   Relation between sexual behaviour and determination of site.

> He came in, noticing me as he entered and stopped about 15 metres away. He stood facing me, rubbing his crotch while looking at me. (Field notes, Railway Sidings)

> A stopped just past the turn in the path and turned around. He walked back down towards B. As he approached B, he rubbed his crotch, stopped and went down the embankment in front of B. When he got to the bottom, he turned back to look at B, took his penis out and started masturbating. (Field notes, Railway Sidings)

Sites do not merely belong to one extreme or the other; they cover a spectrum from the highly socially predetermined to non-places. We can, however, make general inferences that the more the site is integrated with other social or civic uses, the more likely the cruising behaviour will be formulaic and scripted.

The extents to which a site is socially and spatially predetermined also influenced the numbers of men engaging in sexual activities and the types of sexual interactions that occurred (Figure 8.2). The spatial predetermination of most sites tended to facilitate exhibitionistic and voyeuristic sex while prohibiting sex which involved prolonged bodily contact. And when contact sex did occur, the predetermined nature of the sites tended to restrict it to sexual dyads; the more men involved, the greater the contravention of those determinants. The situation was different in sites with little or no spatial or social predetermination (e.g. the Railway Sidings).

Because the site was in no way predetermined, all types and combinations of sexual activity were allowed:

> Two guys fucking almost right against the fence. There were three or four guys standing around watching. (Field notes, Railway Sidings)

> There was four guys standing by the railway tracks against the railings – two couples having sex with each other a little distance away from each other. Me and two others kept walking up and down by them. They were clearly very available as they kept looking at us, but not aggressively and liked the fact that we were watching. It was clear

that they would take on whoever was going to come along. Then one of the other guys edged towards them and joined in. The threesome stayed there for a while. I walked out of the way about 10 feet away to observe. Then three guys kind of came out on to the main path and started standing around there. After a few minutes, they were masturbating also. (Field notes, Railway Sidings)

Sex on PSEs is by no means exclusively voyeuristic or limited to masturbation and fellatio. Generally speaking, the more an interaction progressed from definition through to interest and on to sexual contact, the less formulaic and scripted the forms of communication became. Within sites which were highly predetermined, the sexual act itself never took place under the eyes of the site users, and for the most part it was also hidden from other cruisers and cottagers:

When I went in there was no one there. I stood at the urinal. I stood there for a good ten minutes without anyone coming into the cottage. Finally a guy wearing tracksuit pants came in and stood about three urinals away from me. I thought that he was straight, so I assumed a position of legitimacy and acted as if I was just finishing a pee. As I stood away from the urinal, I saw that another guy had also come in and was standing two urinals away from him. I went into the wash-room and stood just behind the doorway. I could see the guy who came in last. He was gay-looking and was watching the tracksuit guy who was standing two urinals away. He also turned to look at me; however, his look was simply to see if I was watching. He did not appear to be interested in me at all. After a couple of minutes another person came into the cottage and went into a cubicle. As he came in I moved further into the washroom. After I heard the door of the cubicle close, I went back to the doorway. I looked around and saw the two guys from the urinals go into a cubicle. They had left the door open and the tracksuit guy was standing almost in the doorway of the cubicle, looking out every now and then to see if the coast was clear. I stood there for about ten minutes when I saw the two guys leave separately. (Field notes, Mill Street Cottage)

To understand how sexual behaviour (as opposed to cruising behaviour) is likely to be influenced by the nature of the site, one must first understand the importance of the negotiation of risk between users of that site. Within sites which are both highly socially and spatially predetermined, it is generally true that the closer the physical contact achieved, the greater the contravention of social norms. However, this is by no means always the case. Certain sites (e.g. public toilets) are often spatially determined in order to allow for relations of proximity to be achieved between users, and these relations allow them to engage in sexual contact without contravening the socially predetermined

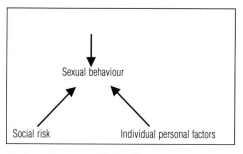

Figure 8.3   Factors influencing sexual behaviour.

norms (e.g. sexual contact at the urinals of a cottage, or between the urinals and a cubicle). Other sites, however, offer 'pockets' of privacy in which full physical contact can take place (e.g. the bushy areas between the paths at Avon Cemetery).

Notwithstanding this, all sexual encounters in PSEs run the risk of interruption and exposure (Figure 8.3). In some sites the risk is greater than others. However, all sites have the capacity for men to take as much risk as they want. Therefore, in certain cottages, it will be extremely rare for two men to have sex in a cubicle whereas in others it will not. The extent to which men risk exposure is a personal choice, but the social and spatial predetermination of that site will inevitably influence how great is the risk perceived. Therefore, to engage in sex with another man in the locked cubicle of a toilet in the middle of a deserted park on a December afternoon will be perceived as less risky than the same actions in a cottage on a busy high street at lunch time. However, much of the movement we have witnessed of men around a site once mutual interest has been established seems likely to be negotiation of how close men are going to get to each other in what area of the site.

The type of sex that occurs in PSEs therefore depends upon the complex interactions of a range of factors. This chapter has attempted to identify and explain them. The type of sex in which participants are going to engage is informed by an interaction between (a) how the site is predetermined socially and spatially and (b) the willingness of couples to take specifically social as opposed to sexual risks. This in turn is most likely influenced by a range of personal factors concerned with sexual desire, past experience, etc. It is not the case that some or any sites prohibit entirely the occurrence of certain forms of sex, rather sites will to a greater or lesser extent discourage certain sexual interactions. However, we can construct a schema for assessing the likelihood of intimate sexual activity involving prolonged bodily contact occurring on any site. What is significant in this assessment is how those aspects which predetermine the site (proximity, access and privacy) coalesce to form an index of greater or lesser risk within which cruisers or cottagers operate. The nature of their social and sexual interaction is determined by this index as well as factors personal to them. Certain sites by their nature will definitely inhibit certain forms of sexual behaviour and it is possible to determine which sites these are.

References

AGGLETON, P. *et al.* (1992) *Outreach Work with Men who Have Sex with Men.* Report from a national consultation on outreach and detached work with men who have sex with men. Bristol: Southmead Health Authority.

BELL, A.P. and WEINBERG, M.S. (1978) *Homosexualities: A Study of Diversity Among Men and Women.* London: Mitchell Beazley.

BURGESS, R. (1991) *In the Field: An Introduction to Field Research.* London: Routledge.

CHURCH, J., GREEN, J., VERNEALS, S. and KEOGH, P. (1993) 'Investigation of motivational and behavioural factors influencing men who have sex with men in public toilets (cottaging)', *AIDS Care*, **5**, 3, pp. 337–46.

DELPH, E. (1978) *The Silent Community.* London: Sage.

HUMPHREYS, L. (1970) *Tearoom Trade.* London: Duckworth.

KEOGH, P., HOLLAND, P. and WEATHERBURN, P. (1998) *The Boys in the Backroom: Anonymous Sex Among Gay and Bisexual Men.* Report to the Inner London HIV Health Commissioners Group. London: Sigma Research.

KEOGH, P., GREEN, J., VERNEALS, S. and CHURCH, J. (1993) 'Motivational and behavioural factors influencing men who cruise in the United Kingdom'. Poster presentation for the IXth International AIDS Conference, Berlin (PO-DO6-3590).

LOFTLAND, J. and LOFTLAND, L. (1995) *Analysing Social Settings.* Vermont: Wadsworth.

PONTE, M.R. (1974) 'Life in parking lot: an ethnography of a homosexual drive-in', in Jacobs, J. (ed.) *Deviance: Field Studies and Self Disclosures.* Palo Alto, CA: National Press Books.

STYLES, J. (1979) 'Outsider/insider: researching gay baths', *Urban Life*, **8**, pp. 135–52.

WEATHERBURN, P. *et al.* (1996) *Behaviourally Bisexual Men in the UK: Identifying Needs for HIV Prevention.* Commissioned report for the Health Education Authority. London: Sigma Research.

ZNANIECKI, F. (1934) *The Method of Sociology.* New York: Farrar and Rienhart.

Chapter 9

Sydney Gay Men's Agreements about Sex

Paul Van de Ven, Judy French, June Crawford and Susan Kippax

At a time of increasingly complex HIV/AIDS issues, we set out to examine gay men's agreements and practices in relation to anal intercourse with their regular partners and involvement with casual partners. It has been argued that patterns of gay male sexual practice have evolved with the HIV epidemic and that gay men have gradually adopted new and more sophisticated personal strategies of safe sex. Gay men are changing their risk practices in response to the cumulative impact of the epidemic, and they continually balance their risk of infection with other personal needs (Kinder, 1996). One of the emerging trends is the negotiation of 'safe' unprotected anal intercourse within relationships.

It is well documented that awareness of concordant HIV negative status, particularly in ongoing partnerships, is associated with gay men's engagement in unprotected anal intercourse, (Bosga *et al.*, 1995; Dawson *et al.*, 1994; Detels *et al.*, 1989; Kippax, 1996; Ridge, Plummer and Minichiello, 1994). At the beginning of the decade, this phenomenon was taken to indicate that gay men were 'relapsing to unsafe sex' (Adib *et al.*, 1991; Stall *et al.*, 1990). It sparked a debate between those that would characterize gay men who engage in unprotected anal intercourse as individually deficient, irresponsible and feckless and those that would want to explore the context and interpersonal dynamics of what may be a rational decision and a safe interaction (Davies and Project SIGMA, 1992).

In earlier work (Kippax *et al.*, 1993) it was demonstrated that the majority of gay men negotiate their sexual activity. Within their regular relationships, 79% of men had a 'clear agreement' on sexual practice. Most (82%) of those who agreed that anal intercourse could take place without a condom were in concordant (positive–positive or negative–negative) relationships, and 80% reported never having broken the agreement. Correspondingly, for sexual involvement outside their regular relationships, 74% of men had a 'clear agreement' (39% had no casual sex; 36% had protected sex both inside and outside the relationship; 23% had protected sex with casual partners only) and 81% reported never having broken the agreement.

In a more recent analysis of sexual negotiations (Kippax *et al.*, 1997) it was found that 61.9% of 181 men in concordant negative relationships of six months duration or longer engaged in unprotected anal intercourse (at least once in the six months prior to interview) with their regular partner. Of these 181 men, 80% had an agreement with their regular partner about the nature of their involvement with casual partners. The presence of such an agreement was predictive of safe sex when compared with no agreement at all. Moreover, the best agreement with regard to safe casual sex was 'casual sex but no anal sex', for men who had this type of agreement tended not to engage in unprotected anal intercourse with casual partners.

Previously, comprehensive analyses of sex agreements and subsequent sexual practices have been problematic because the large sample sizes required to analyze gay men's agreements under various circumstances were not available. For example, it is argued that agreements should be assessed separately for men in regular relationships which, in terms of the partners' HIV statuses, can be concordant (both partners negative or both positive), discordant (partners of known opposite status) or non-concordant (one or both partners of unknown status, either untested or undisclosed). Separate analyses for each of the three serostatus combinations are appropriate because of the different meanings and motivations associated with agreements in these different types of relationship.

Furthermore, it is necessary to limit analyses of agreements and practices to men who have been in a regular relationship for at least six months. Only by doing so can agreements with a 'current' regular partner be assessed against relevant sexual practices in the six months prior to data collection. That is, the sexual practice data necessarily pertain wholly to the current regular partner and, if applicable, the current agreement.

The Sydney Gay Community Periodic Survey conducted in February 1996 had 1,611 respondents. This large database was suitable for a thorough analysis of agreements and sexual practices. Apart from a general mapping of the field of sex agreements and associated practice, we were also keen to explore the terrain around concordant-negative relationships. Of particular interest were men in concordant-negative relationships who had 'negotiated safety' agreements that permitted unprotected anal intercourse within their relationships but only 'safe' involvements with casual partners. Argued in terms of unprotected anal intercourse with casual partners, two questions of interest were: How well do negotiated safety agreements fare and are some types of agreement about casual sex more protective than others?

Methodology

Participants

Study participants were gay and homosexually active men who attended either the Gay and Lesbian Mardi Gras Fair Day on Sunday 11 February 1996, or one of six venues during the subsequent week. Two of the venues were sexual health clinics; the other four (a sauna, a sex club, a gay bar and a sports venue) were gay venues in both inner and outer suburban Sydney. Men were included in the survey if they had had sex with another man in the past five years *and* they lived in Sydney or participated regularly in Sydney gay community *and* they had not completed the survey elsewhere during the week.

Questionnaire

An anonymous, self-completed questionnaire was used. The two-page (single-sheet) instrument took approximately five minutes to complete. Items covered some demographics, aspects of gay community attachment, sexual identity, sexual relationships and agreements, sexual practices with men and with women, and HIV testing and results. The use of these types of questions and instruments has been validated by way of triangulation in previous studies of gay men.

Two specific questions about sex agreements were asked. Concerning regular partners, men were asked, Do you have a clear (spoken) agreement with your regular partner about anal sex (fucking) *within your relationship*? The men chose one of four response categories:

- No agreement
- Agreement: no anal sex at all
- Agreement: all anal sex is with a condom
- Agreement: anal sex can be without a condom

Concerning casual partners, men were asked, Do you have a clear (spoken) agreement with your regular partner about sex *with casual partners*? The men chose one of five response categories:

- No agreement
- Agreement: no sex at all
- Agreement: no anal sex at all
- Agreement: all anal sex is with a condom
- Agreement: anal sex can be without a condom

Procedure

As well as the Gay and Lesbian Mardi Gras Fair Day, six diverse venues frequented by men were selected to attain the most inclusive sample of Sydney's homosexually active men. The fair day and the venues were chosen by a large group of researchers, health practitioners and gay educators, some of them gay men, based on long-standing personal and professional knowledge of Sydney's gay community. Two sexual health clinics (one inner-city, one suburban) were included to ensure representation in the overall sample of

HIV positive men and of those at higher risk of STD infection. Each of the venue managers agreed to cooperate in the survey. As a first step, the questionnaire was pilot-tested at one of the gay venues and subsequently amended to eliminate ambiguities.

A combination of paid and volunteer recruiters, as well as venue staff, was used for recruitment. Recruiters were trained in the application of a standardized procedure. All men attending the venues were approached. At the fair day, recruiters were positioned at strategic stalls and alleyways and they approached as many men as possible. Most participants were recruited personally. At venues with extended opening hours, it was possible for men to complete a questionnaire in the absence of recruiters. An initial comparison of the responses of men who completed a questionnaire in the absence of a recruiter ($n = 73$) with the others' responses revealed no substantial differences attributable to presence of a recruiter.

Participation was voluntary. However, to encourage participation at the Gay and Lesbian Mardi Gras Fair Day, men who returned a completed questionnaire to a 'ballot box' were offered the opportunity to enter a draw. The prize was a dinner for two at one of Sydney's leading restaurants, and it was donated by the restaurateur.

Data Analysis

The data was analyzed by venue and as a whole. There were no significant differences between the venues in respect of the participants' ethnocultural backgrounds and lengths of relationships, as well as most of their sexual practices with men and with women. In separate analyses (not reported here) we found some differences between the various clinic and venue samples, but there was no evidence to suggest these differences would confound the results presented here. Hence, in the interests of a more inclusive picture, the findings reported here are based on the data set in its entirety.

The analysis of agreements about sex was limited to men who had been in a regular relationship for six months or longer. This was done to ensure that the agreements the men reported applied to their current relationship and that those agreements could be assessed against questions about sexual practice with regular and casual partners 'in the past six months'.

Results

The total number of participants was 1,611 men; this represents a recruiter response rate of 84.1%. Of 1,828 men approached, 290 refused to participate. However, there was no way of measuring non-response in recruiter absence. Most of the men ($n = 1,034$) were recruited at the Gay and Lesbian Mardi Gras Fair Day, with 336 recruited at the gay venues and 241 at the sexual health clinics.

Demographics and Milieu

The demographic characteristics of the sample were essentially similar to samples in other large-scale studies of gay men (Prestage *et al.*, 1995). The 1,611 participants ranged in age from 17 to 72 years (median 34). In terms of ethnocultural background, 84.2% described themselves as Anglo-Australian, and 7.3% and 8.5% were of European and non-European background, respectively. Most of the men lived in inner Sydney (28.7%), the gay districts of Sydney (22.2%), or the nearby eastern suburbs (16.8%). The others lived in outer suburban areas of Sydney.

Overall, almost half of the men (46.7%) had attended a tertiary educational institution. About two-thirds of the men (64.6%) worked for a salary, while 16.6% were self-employed. Approximately half of the participants (49.5%) occupied managerial or professional positions. The remainder were in clerical or sales (24.9%), paraprofessional (13.1%), trade (9.3%) or plant operator/labouring (3.2%) roles.

The sample as a whole had quite firm attachment to gay community. Almost two-thirds of the men (63.8%) indicated that most or all of their friends were gay or homosexual men. Likewise, more than half of the men (57.8%) said that they spent 'a lot' of their free time with other gay or homosexual men. Most of the men (86.0%) had tested for HIV and over two-thirds (70.0%) had done so in the previous twelve months. For the group as a whole, 17.0% were HIV positive, 68.8% HIV negative, and 11.2% untested (missing data accounted for 3.0%).

Sexual Identity and Relations

Most of the men (91.2%) identified as gay or homosexual, rather than as bisexual or heterosexual. Corresponding with their gay identification, the men chiefly enjoyed having sex with 'men only' (84.1%) or 'mostly men' (11.9%). The modal range for number of male sex partners 'in the previous six months' (collapsed categories: none, one, 2–10, 11–50, >50) was 2 to 10 men (42.6%). Few men (5.1%) had more than 50 male sex partners in that period. And most of the participants (92.4%) had no female sex partners in the six months prior to the survey. Forty-five men had regular female sex partners, 55 had casual female partners and 14 had both regular and casual female partners.

At the survey time and for the sample as a whole, relationships with men were as follows. Some 27.0% of the men were in a monogamous regular relationship, 36.3% were in a regular relationship where either or both partners also had casual sexual partners, and 23.1% had casual sex only. The other men (13.5%) stated they were not involved in any sexual relations with men at that time.

The remaining analyses were limited to men who had been in a regular relationship for more than six months. There were 716 such participants

Table 9.1 Men who have been in a regular relationship for more than six months ($n = 716$)

Duration	n	%
6–11 months	108	15.1
1–2 years	194	27.1
3–5 years	183	25.6
>5 years	231	32.3

Table 9.2 Participant's HIV status by regular partner's HIV status ($n = 660$)

	Partner's HIV status		
Participant's HIV status	Positive	Negative	Unknown
Positive	70[a]	50[b]	19[c]
Negative	54[b]	378[a]	46[c]
Unknown	3[c]	25[c]	15[c]

[a] Concordant (67.9%).
[b] Discordant (15.8%).
[c] Non-concordant (16.4%).

and their relationship durations are presented in Table 9.1. The relationships had lasted for varying amounts of time, with almost one-third (32.3%) of this subsample having been in a regular relationship for more than five years.

Table 9.2 shows a participant's HIV status against his regular partner's status, where this information was recorded on the questionnaire. Over two-thirds of the men were in concordant (negative–negative or positive–positive) relationships.

Agreements

Agreements about anal intercourse within the relationship are given in Table 9.3. Unprotected anal intercourse was the most common agreement for men in concordant relationships (48.5%) whereas protected anal intercourse was the most common agreement for those in discordant (62.0%) or non-concordant relationships (37.4%). Few men in discordant relationships (6.0%) agreed to engage in unprotected anal intercourse. A quarter of men in non-concordant relationships (25.2%) agreed on unprotected anal intercourse. Moreover,

Table 9.3   Agreements about anal intercourse within the relationship (%)

	Concordant n = 441	Discordant n = 100	Non-concordant n = 107
No agreement	15.2	16.0	29.0
No anal intercourse	6.6	16.0	8.4
Condoms	29.7	62.0	37.4
No condoms	48.5	6.0	25.2

Table 9.4   Agreements about casual sex (%)

	Concordant n = 429	Discordant n = 95	Non-concordant n = 98
No agreement	24.5	33.7	38.8
No casual partners	28.7	22.1	25.5
No anal intercourse	11.9	5.3	7.1
Condoms	32.6	37.9	27.6
No condoms	2.3	1.1	1.0

those in non-concordant relationships were the most likely to report 'no agreement' (29.0%).

Agreements about casual sex are presented in Table 9.4. Men in concordant and discordant relationships most commonly agreed on protected anal intercourse with casual partners, but those in non-concordant relationships most commonly had no agreement about casual partners. About a quarter of the men in each of the three serostatus combinations had agreed to have no casual sex partners. Relatively few men had struck an agreement to engage in no anal intercourse with casual partners, and very few had settled on unprotected anal intercourse with casual partners.

Agreements and Practice

Table 9.5 sets out the men's reported sexual practice 'in the previous six months' with their regular partners, against their agreements and for each serostatus combination. Practice was predominantly in line with agreements, regardless of serostatus combination, and particularly for the men who had agreed on 'condoms always' or 'no condoms'. For the men who had no agreement in concordant and non-concordant regular relationships, 'any unprotected anal intercourse' most commonly occurred. For their discordant

Table 9.5 Anal intercourse between regular partners 'in the previous six months' by sex agreements (%)

	No anal intercourse	100% protected anal intercourse	Any unprotected anal intercourse
CONCORDANT PARTNERS (N = 438)			
No agreement (n = 66)	27.3	15.2	57.6
No anal intercourse (n = 28)	60.7	14.3	25.0
Condoms (n = 131)	13.7	67.2	19.1
No condoms (n = 213)	4.2	5.2	90.6
DISCORDANT PARTNERS (N = 98)			
No agreement (n = 16)	31.3	37.5	31.3
No anal intercourse (n = 14)	78.6	7.1	14.3
Condoms (n = 62)	3.2	80.6	16.1
No condoms (n = 6)	–	–	100.0
NON-CONCORDANT PARTNERS (N = 105)			
No agreement (n = 30)	26.7	23.3	50.0
No anal intercourse (n = 8)	62.5	25.0	12.5
Condoms (n = 40)	7.5	85.0	7.5
No condoms (n = 27)	7.4	11.1	81.5

counterparts, '100% protected anal intercourse' was slightly more common than other practices.

Table 9.6 shows the men's reported involvement 'in the previous six months' with casual partners, against their agreements and for each serostatus combination. Men in concordant regular relationships tended to adhere to their 'safe sex' agreements. Those who had no agreement or who had an 'unsafe sex' agreement were more likely to have had any unprotected anal intercourse with casual partners.

Men in discordant or non-concordant regular relationships tended to adhere to their 'no anal intercourse' and 'condoms' with casual partners agreements. Their counterparts who had agreed on 'no casual partners' tended to end up having casual partners but with whom they typically did not have anal intercourse. The other men who had no agreement usually reported having casual partners with whom they most commonly had no anal intercourse or protected anal intercourse only.

Generally, the men who reported having the least unprotected anal intercourse with casual partners were those who had agreed to engage in sex with casual partners, but such sex was not to include anal intercourse. For most of these men, involvement with casual partners resulted in safe outcomes, for where they slipped up they tended to engage in '100% protected anal intercourse'.

Table 9.6 Involvement with casual partners 'in the previous six months' by seroconcordance in regular relationship and agreements about casual sex (%)

	No casual partners	No anal intercourse	100% protected anal intercourse	Any unprotected anal intercourse
CONCORDANT (*N* = 426)				
No agreement (*n* = 104)	26.9	35.6	16.3	21.2
No casual partners (*n* = 123)	51.2	37.4	5.7	5.7
No anal intercourse (*n* = 51)	13.7	56.9	25.5	3.9
Condoms (*n* = 138)	5.8	23.2	63.0	8.0
No condoms (*n* = 10)	30.0	20.0	20.0	30.0
DISCORDANT (*N* = 94)				
No agreement (*n* = 31)	19.4	35.5	32.3	12.9
No casual partners (*n* = 21)	38.1	52.4	4.8	4.8
No anal intercourse (*n* = 5)	40.0	40.0	20.0	–
Condoms (*n* = 36)	13.9	22.2	50.0	13.9
No condoms (*n* = 1)	–	–	100.0	–
NON-CONCORDANT (*N* = 96)				
No agreement (*n* = 36)	16.7	38.9	33.3	11.1
No casual partners (*n* = 25)	40.0	52.0	4.0	4.0
No anal intercourse (*n* = 7)	14.3	57.1	28.6	–
Condoms (*n* = 27)	3.7	25.9	70.4	–
No condoms (*n* = 1)	–	–	–	100.0

Concordant-Negative Relationships

Data was available on 378 men who had been in a concordant-negative regular relationship of greater than six months duration. The lengths of these men's relationships are given in Table 9.7.

For the men in concordant-negative relationships, agreements about anal intercourse within the relationship and about casual sex are presented in Table 9.8. 'No condoms' was the most common agreement within a relationship (47.5%). The men had a variety of agreements about involvement with casual partners. About a quarter of the men (24.7%) had no casual partner agreement, and very few agreed that anal intercourse with casual partners could be without condoms (1.9%).

Negotiated Safety

In all, 142 of the men in concordant-negative relationships (37.6% of this select subgroup) had a negotiated safety agreement. That is, they agreed on

Table 9.7 Length of relationships for men in concordant-negative relationships of longer than six months duration ($n = 378$)

Duration	n	%
6–11 months	49	13.0
1–2 years	103	27.2
3–5 years	103	27.2
>5 years	123	32.5

Table 9.8 Men in concordant-negative relationships: agreements about anal intercourse within the relationship and about casual sex

	n	%
WITHIN THE RELATIONSHIP ($N = 373$)		
No agreement	54	14.5
No anal intercourse	24	6.4
Condoms	118	31.6
No condoms	177	47.5
ABOUT CASUAL SEX ($N = 361$)		
No agreement	89	24.7
No casual partners	113	31.3
No anal intercourse	45	12.5
Condoms	107	29.6
No condoms	7	1.9

'no condoms' within the relationship *and* they had an agreement about 'safe' casual sex (not 'no condoms'). So 236 (62.4%) men who *could* have a negotiated safety agreement did not have one.

For the men in these concordant-negative 'negotiated safety' relationships, anal intercourse within the relationship 'in the previous six months' is presented in Table 9.9. Most of these men (90.1%) had instances of unprotected anal intercourse with their regular partners.

For the men in concordant-negative 'negotiated safety' relationships, reported involvement with casual partners 'in the previous six months' is presented against casual sex agreements in Table 9.10. For the men who had agreed on 'no anal intercourse' or 'condoms always' with casual partners, practice tended to be in line with agreements and resulted in few instances of unprotected anal intercourse with casual partners (8.7% and 6.0%, respectively). Likewise, for those who had agreed not to have casual sex, there were

Table 9.9 Men in 'negotiated safety' relationships: anal intercourse within the relationship 'in the previous six months' ($n = 141$)

	n	%
No anal intercourse	6	4.3
100% protected anal intercourse	8	5.7
Any unprotected anal intercourse	127	90.1

Table 9.10 Men in 'negotiated safety' relationships: involvement with casual partners 'in the previous six months' by sex agreements ($n = 142$)

	Involvement with casual partners							
	No casual partners		No anal intercourse		100% protected anal intercourse		Any unprotected anal intercourse	
Agreement	n	%	n	%	n	%	n	%
No casual partners	32	46.4	29	42.0	4	5.8	4	5.8
No anal intercourse	2	8.7	14	60.9	5	21.7	2	8.7
Condoms	3	6.0	11	22.0	33	66.0	3	6.0

few instances of unprotected anal intercourse with casual partners (5.8%). However, for this latter group of men, having casual sex but without anal intercourse (42.0%) was about as likely as adhering to the agreement not to have casual sex (46.4%).

Discussion

Our data, drawn from a sample of 1,611 gay men and based on 716 who had been in a regular relationship for more than six months, shows that gay men tend to have agreements with their regular partners about sex within and outside their relationships. The types of agreement they have vary somewhat according to the serostatus combination in their regular relationship. For men in concordant relationships, unprotected anal intercourse within the relationship was the most common agreement. For those in discordant or non-concordant relationships, as was to be expected, protected anal intercourse within the relationship was the most common agreement. Men in concordant and discordant relationships most commonly agreed on protected anal inter-course with casual partners whereas those in non-concordant relationships most commonly had no agreement about casual partners.

Men who had agreements about anal intercourse within the relationship tended to adhere to their agreements in practice. Those who had no agreement most commonly ended up having instances of unprotected anal intercourse within concordant or non-concordant relationships, rather less so within discordant relationships. Men who had agreements about 'safe' involvement with casual partners (either 'no anal intercourse' or 'condoms always') tended to stick to their agreements. Importantly, men in concordant or non-concord-ant relationships who had no agreement about sex outside their relationships were more likely to report instances of unprotected anal intercourse with casual partners.

Of those in concordant-negative relationships that were of greater than six months duration, 142 men had a negotiated safety agreement of 'no condoms' within the relationship coupled with 'no casual sex', 'no casual anal intercourse' or 'condoms always with casual partners'. For these men, practice tended to be in line with agreements and resulted in few instances of unpro-tected anal intercourse with casual partners. Unlike an earlier finding based on a different Sydney sample in which an agreement to have casual sex but no casual anal intercourse was the best agreement (Kippax *et al.*, 1997), in this analysis, no one type of 'casual sex' agreement was better in terms of avoidance of unprotected anal intercourse with casual partners. In sum, measured against instances of unprotected anal intercourse with casual partners, negotiated safety agreements seem to perform fairly well regardless of the specific type of agreement about casual sex.

In terms of risk of HIV transmission, having 'safe sex' agreements is generally more protective than not having agreements. Men in discordant or non-concordant relationships who have not reached agreement about sex within their relationships are much more likely to have unprotected anal intercourse with their regular partners than those with a 'safe sex' agreement. Likewise, regardless of the serostatus combination within the regular relation-ship, those *without* agreements about 'casual sex' are generally more likely to engage in unprotected anal intercourse with casual partners. Furthermore, very few men in concordant-negative relationships practising 'negotiated safety' end up having unprotected anal intercourse with casual partners. These are key messages for HIV educators, especially those responsible for educat-ing about safe unprotected anal intercourse within relationships.

Why should it be that 'safe sex' agreements are protective? Is it simply that once men have consented to do something, they avoid dissonance and going back on their word so as not to deceive their partners? This is perhaps only partially responsible for the protective value of agreements. It is more likely to be the case that relationships in which agreements are reached are characterized by a certain openness, with good communication and mutual respect and trust. The challenge for sexual health education programmes is to explore ways to help gay men develop their relationships in the direction of sound communication, acceptance and shared trust. Part of this process must include providing partners with reliable and supportive strategies for reporting and dealing with breaches of the agreements, particularly where they involve unprotected anal intercourse with casual partners, for our data reveals that such lapses do occur. Unless these lapses can be communicated and handled in an atmosphere free from rancour, recrimination and retribution, the entire case for negotiating sexual safety through agreements is in jeopardy.

Now it will also be necessary to analyse agreements and sexual practices in light of viral load testing and combination HIV therapies. Part of gay men's evolving response to the epidemic – at a time distinguished by the emergence of new and promising health management options – may be to incorporate results of viral load tests and changes in health and well-being following combination therapy into decisions and agreements about sex with regular and casual partners. Little so far is known about the extent or efficacy of these strategies. What is certain, though, is that we are living in a different era from the one in which to slip on a condom every time seemed such a sensible, indeed the only rational, way to requite gay men's desire for anal intercourse while avoiding HIV transmission.

Acknowledgement

The Sydney Gay Community Periodic Survey was a joint research project of the National Centre in HIV Social Research (Macquarie University), the National Centre in HIV Epidemiology and Clinical Research (University of New South Wales) and the AIDS Council of New South Wales. The project was supported by the AIDS/Infectious Diseases Branch, New South Wales Health Department.

References

ADIB, S.M., JOSEPH, J.G., OSTROW, D.G., TAL, M. and SCHWARTZ, S.M. (1991) 'Relapse in sexual behaviour among homosexual men: a two-year follow-up from the Chicago MACS/CCS', *AIDS*, **5**, pp. 757–60.

BOSGA, M.B., DE WIT, J.B.F., DE VROOME, E.M.M., HOUWELING, H., SCHOP, W. and SANDFORT, T.G.M. (1995) 'Differences in perception of risk for HIV infection with steady and non-steady partners among homosexual men', *AIDS Education and Prevention*, **7**, pp. 103–15.

DAVIES, P. and PROJECT SIGMA. (1992) 'On relapse: recidivism or rational response?', in Aggleton, P., Davies, P. and Hart, G. (eds) *AIDS: Rights, Risk and Reason*. London: Falmer Press.

DAWSON, J.M., FITZPATRICK, R.M., REEVES, G., BOULTON, M., McLEAN, J., HART, G.J. and BROOKES, M. (1994) 'Awareness of sexual partners' HIV status as an influence upon high-risk sexual behaviour among gay men', *AIDS*, **8**, pp. 837–41.

DETELS, R., ENGLISH, P., VISSCHER, B.R., JACOBSON, L., KINGSLEY, L.A., CHMIEL, J.S., DUDLEY, J.P., ELDRED, L.J. and GINZBURG, H.M. (1989) 'Seroconversion, sexual activity and condom use among 2915 HIV seronegative men followed for up to 2 years', *Journal of Acquired Immunodeficiency Syndrome*, **2**, pp. 77–83.

KINDER, P. (1996) 'A new prevention education strategy for gay men: responding to the impact of AIDS in gay men's lives'. Paper given at the XIth International Conference on AIDS, Vancouver.

KIPPAX, S. (1996) 'A commentary on negotiated safety', *Venereology*, **9**, pp. 96–97.

KIPPAX, S., CRAWFORD, J., DAVIS, M., RODDEN, P. and DOWSETT, G. (1993) 'Sustaining safe sex: a longitudinal study of a sample of homosexual men', *AIDS*, **7**, pp. 257–63.

KIPPAX, S., NOBLE, J., PRESTAGE, G., CRAWFORD, J., CAMPBELL, D., BAXTER, D. and COOPER, D. (1997) 'Sexual negotiation in the AIDS era: negotiated safety revisited', *AIDS*, **11**, pp. 191–97.

PRESTAGE, G., NOBLE, J., KIPPAX, S., CRAWFORD, J., BAXTER, D. and COOPER, D. (1995) *Methods and Sample in a Study of Homosexually-active Men in Sydney, Australia*. Sydney: HIV, AIDS and Society Publications.

RIDGE, D.T., PLUMMER, D.C. and MINICHIELLO, V. (1994) 'Knowledge and practice of sexual safety in Melbourne gay men in the nineties', *Australian Journal of Public Health*, **18**, pp. 310–25.

STALL, R.D., EKSTRAND, M., POLLACK, L., McKUSICK, L. and COATES, T. (1990) 'Relapse to unsafe sex: the next challenge for AIDS prevention efforts', *Journal of Acquired Immunodeficiency Syndrome*, **3**, pp. 1181–87.

Chapter 10

Young Gay Men and HIV Risk

Danielle Campbell, Paul Van de Ven, Garrett Prestage,
June Crawford and Susan Kippax

At the XIth International Conference on AIDS in Vancouver, de Wit (1996a) presented a critique of the present literature pertaining to young gay men and HIV/AIDS. The studies reviewed by de Wit (1996a; 1996b) provided evidence for increased HIV risk among gay youth. Yet, as both Flowers (1997) and Van de Ven *et al.* (1998) have noted, the relationship between youth and elevated risk of HIV is not universal, and studies of young gay men and sexual risk have produced mixed findings.

Since the late 1980s, several North American studies have reported an association between younger age and risky sexual behaviour in cohorts of gay men (e.g. Ekstrand and Coates, 1990; Hays, Kegeles and Coates, 1990; Kelly *et al.*, 1990, 1995; McCusick *et al.*, 1990; Morris, Zavisca and Dean, 1995; Stall *et al.*, 1992; Valdiserri *et al.*, 1988). Data from Canada (Myers *et al.*, 1992), Amsterdam (de Wit and van Griensven, 1994) and Denmark (Schmidt *et al.*, 1992) has conformed to this pattern of results. Young gay men's alleged propensity for sexual risk taking has been variously attributed to a developmental inclination toward risk taking and impulsivity in general (Ekstrand and Coates, 1990; Hays, Kegeles and Coates, 1990; Schmidt *et al.*, 1992; Stall *et al.*, 1992); illusions of invulnerability (Ekstrand and Coates, 1990; Hays, Kegeles and Coates, 1990); feelings of isolation and alienation associated with a lack of social support networks (Ekstrand and Coates, 1990; Hays, Kegeles and Coates, 1990); and poor communication and safe sex negotiation skills (Ekstrand and Coates, 1990; Hays, Kegeles and Coates, 1990; Schmidt *et al.*, 1992).

In contrast to findings from these North American and continental European studies, Davies *et al.* (1992) found that English and Welsh gay men under 21 years of age used condoms slightly more consistently than their older counterparts, and were as knowledgeable as the older gay men about HIV risk and safer sex. Results from various Australian studies are comparable. In an early study of gay men and sexual practice in New South Wales, Connell *et al.* (1990) reported that men aged under 25 years were least likely to have unprotected anal intercourse with regular partners, and that unprotected anal intercourse with casual partners was independent of age group. Similarly, in a 1990 Melbourne study there was no difference in the levels of recent unprotected anal intercourse between men under 25 years of age and men aged 25 years and over (Ridge, Plummer and Minichiello, 1994). A nationwide study of homosexually active men interviewed in 1992 also found no significant differences between age groups with regard to condom use with casual partners (Kippax *et al.*, 1994). More recently, two separate Sydney studies of primarily gay-identified and gay-community-attached men (Van de Ven *et al.*, 1997; Van de Ven *et al.*, 1998) have compared the HIV risk behaviours of gay men under the age of 25 with those aged 25 and over. In both cohorts, levels of unprotected anal intercourse with regular and casual male partners were independent of age group, providing further evidence of precautionary sexual behaviour among young Australian gay men.

Commentators have pointed out that while discrepancies between studies of gay youth and sexual risk may be due to substantive intercountry differences, inherent methodological problems and differences between study designs may also be important (Davies *et al.*, 1992; Ridge, Plummer and Minichiello, 1994; Van de Ven *et al.*, 1998). Perhaps the most important of these differences relates to the defining of key concepts. Definitions of youth have ranged from under 21 years (Davies *et al.*, 1992) to under 30 years (Stall *et al.*, 1992). Furthermore, definitions of sexual risk behaviours vary widely across studies and involve diverse distinctions regarding the nature of the sexual relationship (regular or casual), respondent's and partner's HIV status, mode of anal intercourse (insertive or receptive), consistency of condom use, and behavioural time frame. Meyer and Dean (1995) define 'sexual risk behaviour' as acts of receptive anal intercourse with and without condoms in the twelve-month period before interview, whereas Stall *et al.* (1992) define 'high risk' as having engaged in condom-unprotected insertive or receptive anal intercourse outside of a mutually monogamous relationship up to 30 days before interview.

Given this wide variability in definitional and other aspects of study design, it is wise to be cautious over conclusions about increased risk among gay youth which are based on comparing findings from different studies (Davies *et al.*, 1992). Moreover, the growing number of studies which have reported no age-related distinctions in HIV risk behaviours warrant a radical reconsideration of the 'youth–risk' hypothesis. In particular, the view that risk is a natural and universal characteristic of youth rather than a consequence of distinctive social and cultural factors should be addressed. With that aim, this chapter compares the social characteristics and sexual behaviour of young (age under 25 years) and older (age 25 years and over) gay-identified and gay-community-attached men from three large Australian cities. Consonant with earlier studies of Australian gay men, it was postulated that young men would be as precautionary in their sexual behaviour as older men.

Participants

A total of 1,439 men were interviewed; 734 (51.0%) from Sydney, 406 (28.2%) from Melbourne and 299 (20.8%) from Brisbane. Six men (two from Melbourne and four from Brisbane) did not provide date of birth information, so the sample size for this analysis was reduced to 1,433.

Procedure

The data for this paper is drawn from the Sydney (SMASH), Melbourne (MMASH) and Brisbane Region (BRASH) Men and Sexual Health studies. SMASH is an ongoing, longitudinal study for which participants, who were recruited into the cohort from late 1992, are interviewed annually. The Melbourne (Victoria) and Brisbane (Queensland) arms of the project were one-off studies conducted between October 1995 and March 1996. For each of the three studies, gay and other homosexually active men were recruited from diverse (primarily gay community) sources, and comparable face-to-face structured interview schedules were used. Data was collected on a range of issues, including demographic details, sources of HIV information, sexual identity, relationships and sexual practice with men and women, involvement in gay community, knowledge of HIV transmission, health, drug usage, and relationship to people with HIV or AIDS. To ensure temporal comparability with data from the Melbourne and Brisbane studies, the Sydney data used here comes from interviews conducted in the second half of 1995 and the first half of 1996. Bivariate relationships between age and a range of measures related to HIV transmission risk were examined using chi-square for categorical data and ANOVAs (analysis of variance) for continuous variables.

Results

The ages of the 1,433 participants ranged from 14 to 75 years; the median age was 33 years. Some 254 (17.7%) men were under 25 years of age and 1,179 (82.3%) were aged 25 years or older (Table 10.1). An analysis of city of study by age group indicated that the Brisbane sample contained a larger proportion of younger men than Sydney or Melbourne, ($p < .0001$).

Demographics

The age groups differed in relation to various demographic measures for which an age effect is to be expected (Table 10.2). For instance, young men were less likely to have completed a trade certificate or tertiary education;

Table 10.1 City of residence by age

Study	<25 years n (%)	≥25 years n (%)
Sydney (SMASH)	121 (16.5)	613 (83.5)
Melbourne (MMASH)	55 (13.6)	349 (86.4)
Brisbane (BRASH)	78 (26.4)	217 (73.6)
Total	254 (17.7)	1,179 (82.3)

Table 10.2 Demographic characteristics by age

Variable	<25 years (n = 254) n (%)	≥25 years (n = 1,179) n (%)	χ^2	p
Education			49.0	<.00001
School certificate	59 (23.2)	175 (14.8)		
Higher school certificate	93 (36.6)	253 (21.5)		
Trade certificate	38 (15.0)	244 (10.7)		
University degree	64 (25.2)	507 (43.0)		
Employment[a]			22.4	.00006
Full-time	131 (51.8)	772 (65.5)		
Part-time	38 (15.0)	158 (13.4)		
Unemployed	26 (10.3)	58 (4.9)		
Not in workforce	58 (22.9)	190 (16.1)		
Occupation[b]			64.0	<.00001
Professional / managerial	74 (37.9)	643 (65.1)		
White collar	104 (53.3)	247 (25.0)		
Blue collar	17 (8.7)	97 (9.8)		
HIV status[c]			42.1	<.00001
HIV negative	183 (72.3)	883 (75.3)		
HIV positive	19 (7.5)	196 (16.7)		
Unknown	51 (20.2)	94 (8.0)		

[a] Data on this item was missing for 2 men.
[b] Includes only those men who were in the workforce and who provided occupational information (n = 1,182).
[c] Data on this item was missing for 7 men.

fewer young men were employed full-time, and those young men with jobs were less likely to work in professional or managerial occupations and more likely to be employed in white-collar positions.

HIV status and testing behaviour also significantly differentiated younger men from older men (Table 10.2). One in five men under 25 years had not

Table 10.3   Sexual identity, relationships and gay community involvement by age

Variable	<25 years (n = 254) n (%)	≥25 years (n = 1,179) n (%)	Statistic	p
Sexual identity			$\chi^2 = 12.3$	.006
Gay / queer	172 (67.7)	736 (62.4)		
Homosexual	53 (20.9)	346 (29.3)		
Heterosexual / bisexual	10 (3.9)	51 (4.3)		
Other	19 (7.5)	46 (3.9)		
Relationship type			$\chi^2 = 17.9$	.001
None	35 (13.8)	97 (8.2)		
Casual partners only	108 (42.5)	452 (38.3)		
Regular plus casual	47 (18.5)	342 (29.0)		
Regular partner only	63 (24.8)	274 (23.2)		
Other	1 (0.4)	14 (1.2)		
Length of relationship[a]			$\chi^2 = 47.1$	<.00001
<6 months	50 (45.5)	131 (21.3)		
6–11 months	17 (15.5)	81 (13.1)		
1–2 years	31 (28.2)	146 (23.7)		
≥3 years	12 (10.9)	258 (41.9)		
Feels part of gay community			$\chi^2 = 4.6$	NS
Yes	198 (78.0)	982 (83.3)		
No	34 (13.4)	129 (10.9)		
Unsure	22 (8.7)	68 (5.8)		
Sexual involvement in gay community scale (mean)	3.3	2.9	$F = 11.1$	.0009
Contact with the HIV epidemic scale (mean)	4.1	7.1	$F = 154.7$	<.0001

[a] Includes only those men who were in a regular relationship at the time of interview (n = 726).
NS = not significant.

been tested for HIV antibodies or were awaiting initial test results, compared with one in twelve older men. While around three-quarters of each age cohort had tested HIV negative, proportionately more older men had tested HIV positive.

Sexual Identity, Gay Community Involvement and Relationships

With regard to sexual identity, there were no age differences in heterosexual or bisexual identification. However, older men were more likely to identify as 'homosexual' whereas younger men preferred to identify as 'gay' or 'queer' (Table 10.3). Similar proportions (around 80%) of younger and older men felt

Table 10.4 Beliefs about withdrawal by age and city of residence

Study	Believed withdrawal safe n (%)		χ^2	p
	<25 years	≥25 years		
Sydney (SMASH)	($n = 121$)	($n = 613$)		
	15 (12.4)	49 (8.0)	2.5	NS
Melbourne (MMASH)	($n = 55$)	($n = 349$)		
	4 (7.3)	43 (12.3)	1.2	NS
Brisbane (BRASH)	($n = 78$)	($n = 217$)		
	22 (28.2)	32 (14.7)	6.9	.008

NS = not significant.

themselves to be part of gay community. However, on a scale of sexual involvement in gay community,[1] younger men scored more highly, indicating that they looked for male sex partners at a greater range of gay-oriented venues (e.g. gay bars, dance parties, gay social group events). Not surprisingly, younger men had experienced less contact with the HIV epidemic in terms of knowing people with HIV/AIDS and knowing people who have died following AIDS.[2]

Men were also asked about their relationship status at the time of interview (Table 10.3). Younger men were more likely to report having no current relations with men or casual partnerships only, whereas older men were more likely to report having both regular and casual partners at present. Around a quarter of each age cohort had one regular partner only (i.e. were monogamous at the time of interview). Of those men who had regular partners at interview ($n = 726$), younger men were about twice as likely to be in a relationship of less than six months standing.

HIV-Related Knowledge

As an indicator of knowledge about HIV transmission, men were asked their beliefs about the safety of withdrawal (unprotected anal sex and pulling out before ejaculation). Younger men (16.1%) were more likely than older men (10.5%) to believe in the safety of withdrawal, $\chi^2(1, n = 1,433) = 6.49, p = .01$. This difference, however, was largely attributable to city of residence: younger Brisbane men were almost twice as likely as their older Brisbane counterparts to rate withdrawal as a safe practice (Table 10.4).

Recreational Drug Use

While alcohol consumption[3] was independent of age, the age groups differed in terms of reported recreational drug use[4] (Table 10.5). Scores on a scale

Table 10.5   Recreational drug use by age

Variable	<25 years (n = 254) n (%)	≥25 years (n = 1,179) n (%)	Statistic	p
Alcohol consumption scale (mean)	4.5	4.5	$F = 0.007$	NS
General drug use scale (mean)	7.2	6.0	$F = 7.4$	.007
Drug use during sex with regular partner[a]				
Used amyl	65 (42.2)	272 (38.4)	$\chi^2 = 0.8$	NS
Used other drugs/alcohol	83 (53.9)	316 (44.6)	$\chi^2 = 4.4$	.04
Drug use during sex with casual partner(s)[b]				
Used amyl[c]	92 (45.8)	470 (51.1)	$\chi^2 = 1.9$	NS
Used other drugs/alcohol[d]	108 (53.7)	415 (45.3)	$\chi^2 = 4.7$	.03

[a] Includes only those men who had sexual contact with a regular partner in the previous six months (n = 862).
[b] Includes only those men who had sexual contact with a casual partner in the previous six months (n = 1,126).
[c] Data on this item was missing for 6 men.
[d] Data on this item was missing for 9 men.
NS = not significant.

measuring the frequency of use of ten non-prescription drugs indicated that younger men used a greater range of drugs and/or used them more frequently. The use of amyl nitrite inhalants (poppers) specifically to enhance sexual enjoyment with either regular or casual partners was unrelated to age group. However, the use of other (unspecified) drugs and alcohol during sex did differ according to age: in the six months prior to interview, more younger men than older men had used other drugs and alcohol to enhance sexual pleasure with both regular and casual partners.

Sexual Practice and Importance of Anal Intercourse

In relation to number of male sexual partners reported in the six months prior to interview, there were some relatively small age-related differences (Table 10.6). Younger men were more likely to report having had sex with 10 or fewer partners, while older men were more likely than their younger counterparts to have had between 11 and 50 sexual partners.

Table 10.6 Sexual practice and importance of anal intercourse by age

Variable	<25 years (n = 254) n (%)	≥25 years (n = 1,179) n (%)	Statistic	p
Number of sexual partners[a]			$\chi^2 = 9.8$	.02
None	3 (1.2)	45 (3.8)		
10 or fewer	174 (68.8)	733 (62.2)		
11 to 50	55 (21.7)	327 (27.7)		
More than 50	21 (8.3)	74 (6.3)		
Oral/tactile practices (mean)	5.7	5.6	$F = 4.5$	.03
Anal practices (mean)	4.7	4.4	$F = 2.6$	NS
'Esoteric' practices (mean)	1.2	1.6	$F = 6.6$	.01
Importance of anal sex			$\chi^2 = 8.4$	.01
Very important	31 (12.2)	224 (19.0)		
Reasonably important	99 (39.0)	471 (39.9)		
Not important	124 (48.8)	484 (41.1)		

[a] Data on this item was missing for 1 man.

Three scales[5] were devised to measure the range of oral/tactile, anal and 'esoteric' sexual practices in which men engaged (Table 10.6). While younger men engaged in a slightly greater range of oral/tactile practices and a narrower range of esoteric practices, the anal practices scale did not differentiate between age groups. Younger men were, however, less likely to rate anal intercourse as 'very important' to their sexual repertoire, and almost half of the young men rated anal sex as 'not important'.

Seroconcordance and Anal Intercourse with Regular Partners

Around 60% of each age cohort had had sexual contact with a regular male partner in the six months prior to interview (n = 862). Of these, younger men were more likely to have had regular relationships where seroconcordance was unknown (i.e. where one or both partners did not know their HIV status) (Table 10.7). With regard to mode of anal intercourse, young men were as likely as older men to have engaged in insertive anal sex with their regular partner, but were more likely to have had receptive anal sex. There were no significant differences, however, in the percentages of younger and older men who engaged in unprotected anal intercourse within regular relationships

Table 10.7   Seroconcordance and anal intercourse with regular partner by age

Variable	<25 years (n = 154) n (%)	≥25 years (n = 708) n (%)	χ^2	p
Seroconcordance[a]			15.4	.002
Concordant positive	9 (6.7)	45 (6.9)		
Concordant negative	73 (54.5)	395 (60.3)		
Known discordant	7 (5.2)	84 (12.8)		
Concordance unknown	45 (33.6)	131 (20.0)		
Anal intercourse			4.8	NS
No anal sex	20 (13.0)	146 (20.6)		
Only protected anal sex	51 (33.1)	218 (30.8)		
Some unprotected anal sex	83 (53.9)	344 (48.6)		
Insertive anal intercourse	111 (72.1)	477 (67.4)	1.3	NS
Receptive anal intercourse	113 (73.4)	454 (64.1)	4.8	.03
Frequency of unprotected sex[b]			7.0	.03
Very rarely unprotected	14 (16.9)	27 (7.8)		
Sometimes unprotected	22 (26.5)	84 (24.4)		
Always unprotected	47 (56.6)	233 (67.7)		

[a] Data on this item was missing for 73 men.
[b] Includes only those men who had any unprotected anal intercourse with regular partner (n = 427).
NS = not significant.

(about half of the men with regular partners). For those men who did engage in unprotected sex with their regular partner (n = 427), frequency of unprotected anal sex within the relationship distinguished the two age cohorts: older men were more likely never to use condoms.

Since 'negotiated safety' may have acted as a confounding factor, a further analysis of anal intercourse with regular partners by age group was conducted, controlling for seroconcordance of regular relationships. When only those men in non-concordant relationships (known discordant or concordance unknown) were selected, there was no age effect on safety of anal sex within relationships, $\chi^2(2, n = 267) = 2.61$, $p = .27$. Moreover, when the base was further restricted to include only those men in non-concordant relationships who had anal intercourse with their regular partner, the practice of unprotected anal sex in relationships was again independent of age $\chi^2(1, n = 201) = 2.09$, $p = .15$.

Table 10.8   Anal intercourse with casual partners by age

Variable	<25 years (n = 204) n (%)	≥25 years (n = 922) n (%)	χ^2	p
Anal intercourse			3.0	NS
No anal sex	62 (30.4)	287 (31.1)		
Only protected anal sex	95 (46.6)	470 (51.0)		
Some unprotected anal sex	47 (23.0)	165 (17.9)		
Number of condom-unprotected episodes[a]			0.8	NS
One or a few	39 (83.0)	127 (77.0)		
About half (≥3 partners)	3 (6.4)	13 (7.9)		
Most (≥3 partners)	4 (8.5)	21 (12.7)		
All (≥3 partners)	1 (2.1)	4 (2.4)		

[a] Includes only those men who had any unprotected anal intercourse with casual partners (n = 212).

Anal Intercourse with Casual Partners

About 80% of men in each age group had had sexual contact with a casual male partner in the six months prior to interview (n = 1,126). For those men who had casual partner(s), having engaged in unprotected casual anal sex was independent of age group: around 20% of men with casual partners engaged in some unprotected anal intercourse (Table 10.8). For those who had an episode of unprotected sex, the number of unsafe episodes engaged in with casual partners was also unrelated to age.

Discussion

The findings presented here are clearly at odds with a 'gay youth risk' paradigm. Rather, as hypothesized, young gay men in this three-city sample appear to be as precautionary in their sexual behaviour as their older counterparts. This result is consistent with British data (Davies *et al.*, 1992) and findings from earlier Australian studies (Connell *et al.*, 1990; Kippax *et al.*, 1994; Ridge, Plummer and Minichiello, 1994; Van de Ven *et al.*, 1997, 1998).

Note that the men in this study were mostly gay or homosexually identified, and were generally closely attached to gay community. Van de Ven *et al.* (1998) have noted that a well-developed sense of sexual identity and the existence of organized and supportive gay communities in Australia may account for some of the international disparities between studies of gay youth risk. As such, the results of this study should be generalized only to similar populations; safe sex issues for homosexually active men who do not identify as gay and who feel isolated from urban gay communities may be different.

Many of the age-related differences reported here relate to measures on which an age effect is to be expected, and are not causally associated with risk factors for HIV. For instance, younger men were less likely to have completed their education and, consequently, were less likely to have entered the workforce and to be employed in a professional or managerial occupation. Young men also knew fewer people who were living with HIV or who had died following AIDS. However, the majority of men, regardless of age, self-identified as gay or homosexual and considered themselves to be part of gay community. This seemingly well-developed sense of identity and community is in opposition to contentions that young gay men have less social support for safe sex (Ekstrand and Coates, 1990), feel isolated and alienated, and do not fully identify as gay hence fail to perceive themselves as part of a 'risk group' (Hays, Kegeles and Coates, 1990).

Whereas the safety of sexual practice was independent of age in this cohort, sexual relationships and some measures of sexual practice did differentiate younger men from older men. For example, contrary to previous studies where younger men were more likely to have a regular partner (e.g. Davies *et al.*, 1992), most young men in this cohort had no primary relationship or had casual partners only at the time of interview. While younger men looked for their male sexual partners at a greater range of gay-oriented venues, they were less likely than older men to have had sexual contact with more than ten partners in the six months prior to interview. Men under 25 years of age also engaged in less 'esoteric' sex, the practice of which has been associated with seroconversion among Sydney gay men (Kippax *et al.*, 1998), and were less likely than older men to consider anal sex as very important to their sexual repertoire.

Despite the generally precautionary sexual behaviour of men in this cohort, some age-related differences are cause for concern. First, young men used a greater range of recreational drugs and used them more often. Specifically in the context of sex, young men were more likely to have recently used drugs (excluding amyl) and alcohol to enhance sexual pleasure with both regular and casual partners. While drug use and alcohol consumption during sex have been associated with increased sexual risk behaviour (e.g. Hays, Kegeles and Coates, 1990; Myers *et al.*, 1992; Valdiserri *et al.*, 1988), heightened levels of drug use among young men did not translate into greater risk in this cohort. An earlier Melbourne investigation (Gold and Skinner, 1992) of young gay men's justifications for unsafe sex similarly reported that the degree to which men were intoxicated or 'stoned' during sex did not distinguish between safe and unsafe sexual encounters. Nevertheless, the higher levels of recreational drug use reported by younger men is an important issue from a public health point of view.

Second, believing that unprotected anal intercourse without ejaculation (withdrawal) is safe with regard to HIV transmission was associated with youth. This result, however, was largely attributable to city of residence: Brisbane men in general, and young Brisbane men in particular, were most likely to believe in the safety of withdrawal. The finding of regional differences in safety knowledge has a precedent: Project Male-Call (Kippax *et al.*, 1994) revealed that homosexually active men from Queensland were among the least well informed in a national sample. Regional knowledge differences may be attributable, at least in part, to interstate variability in community-based HIV education programmes. For instance, while the gay men's safe sex campaign materials distributed by the AIDS Council of New South Wales are typically 'clear, concise, explicit and erotic' (Bradford, Kippax and Baxter, 1996: 210), sexually explicit Queensland AIDS Council education campaigns have encountered strong political and mainstream community opposition in that state, to the point where they have been withdrawn from circulation (Boyle and Smith, 1995).

Third, younger men were less likely to have been tested for HIV antibodies and, consequently, were more likely to be in relationships where the seroconcordance was unknown (i.e. where one or both partners did not know their HIV status). Van de Ven and colleagues (Van de Ven *et al.*, 1998) have reported an identical pattern of findings from an earlier investigation of young Sydney gay men, and on the basis of their results have argued for the importance of encouraging young men to be tested for HIV. Issues of testing are particularly important given the apparent short-term and relatively transient nature of some young men's relationships.

The findings presented here are at odds with assertions that young gay men engage in high levels of sexual risk taking. Rather than making universal proclamations of gay youth risk, commentators should recognize the diversity of young gay men's experience (Davies *et al.*, 1992; Kippax and Crawford, 1997; Ridge, Plummer and Minichiello, 1994; Van de Ven *et al.*, 1998). Furthermore, age should not be prioritized in HIV research over other relevant and possibly more pertinent distinctions, such as cultural, social or economic disadvantage.

Notes

1 The *sexual involvement in gay community* scale includes six items about looking for male sexual partners at a variety of gay community venues or events, including gay bars, dance parties and gay social group events. It ranges from 0 to 6 and has a Cronbach's α of .66.

2 *Contact with the HIV epidemic* is a four-item scale which measures the extent to which men know people living with HIV/AIDS and people who have died following AIDS. It has a range of 0 to 12 and a Cronbach's α of .69.

3 *Alcohol consumption* is measured by two items about the frequency of consumption of wine or beer and spirits. Its range is 0 to 14 and its Cronbach's α is .53.

4 *General drug use* is a ten-item scale which includes items about the frequency of use of marijuana, amyl, MDA, ethyl chloride, LSD, speed, cocaine, Ecstasy, ice and Valium. It ranges from 0 to 60 and its Cronbach's α is .78.

5 The *oral/tactile practices* scale includes six items about oral practices (kissing, oral sex, masturbating and sensuous touching) engaged in during the six months prior to interview. It has a range of 0 to 6 and a Cronbach's α of .88. The *anal practices* scale is an eight-point scale which includes items about having engaged in oral–anal contact, anal intercourse (including with-drawal) and anal fingering in the previous six months. It has a range of 0 to 8 and a Cronbach's α of .79. The *esoteric practices* scale includes eight items about the practice of fisting, use of sex toys, sadomasochism and watersports. Its range is 0 to 8 and its Cronbach's α is .81.

References

BOYLE, M. and SMITH, C. (1995) 'Taboo sexualities and the subversion of a safe-sex campaign: discourses in the "Gay Swap Card" debacle'. Paper presented at the 3rd HIV, AIDS and Society Conference, Sydney.

BRADFORD, D., KIPPAX, S. and BAXTER, D. (1996) 'HIV prevention in the community: sexual transmission', *Medical Journal of Australia*, **165**, pp. 210–11.

CONNELL, R.W., CRAWFORD, J., DOWSETT, G.W., KIPPAX, S., SINNOTT, V., RODDEN, P., BERG, R., BAXTER, D. and WATSON, L. (1990) 'Danger and context: unsafe anal sexual practice among homosexual and bisexual men in the AIDS crisis', *Australian and New Zealand Journal of Sociology*, **26**, pp. 187–208.

DAVIES, P.M., WEATHERBURN, P., HUNT, A.J., HICKSON, F.C.I., MCMANUS, T.J. and COXON, A.P.M. (1992) 'The sexual behaviour of young gay men in England and Wales', *AIDS Care*, **4**, pp. 259–72.

EKSTRAND, M.L. and COATES, T.J. (1990) 'Maintenance of safer sexual behaviors and predictors of risky sex: the San Francisco men's health study', *American Journal of Public Health*, **80**, pp. 973–77.

FLOWERS, P. (1997) 'Vancouver conference review: interventions – gay men', *AIDS Care*, **9**, pp. 57–62.

GOLD, R.S. and SKINNER, M.J. (1992) 'Situational factors and thought processes associated with unprotected intercourse in young gay men', *AIDS*, **6**, pp. 1021–30.

HAYS, R.B., KEGELES, S.M. and COATES, T.J. (1990) 'High HIV risk-taking among young gay men', *AIDS*, **4**, pp. 901–7.

KELLY, J.A., ST LAWRENCE, J.S., BRASFIELD, T.L., LEMKE, A., AMIDEI, T., ROFFMAN, R.E., HOOD, H.V., SIMTH, J.E., KILGORE, H. and McNEIL, C., JR (1990) 'Psychological factors that predict AIDS high-risk versus AIDS precautionary behavior', *Journal of Consulting and Clinical Psychology*, **58**, pp. 117–20.

KELLY, J.A., SIKKEMA, K.J., WINETT, R.A., SOLOMON, L.J., ROFFMAN, R.A., HECKMAN, T.G., STEVENSON, L.Y., PERRY, M.J., NORMAN, A.D. and DESIDERATO, L.J. (1995) 'Factors predicting continued high-risk behavior among gay men in small cities: psychological, behavioural and demographic characteristics related to unsafe sex', *Journal of Consulting and Clinical Psychology*, **63**, pp. 101–7.

KIPPAX, S., CAMPBELL, D., VAN DE VEN, P., CRAWFORD, J., PRESTAGE, G., KNOX, S., CULPIN, A., KALDOR, J. and KINDER, P. (1998) 'Cultures of sexual adventurism as markers of HIV seroconversion: a case control study in a cohort of Sydney gay men', *AIDS Care*, **10**, pp. 677–88.

KIPPAX, S. and CRAWFORD, J. (1997) 'Facts and fictions of adolescent risk', in Sherr, L. (ed.) *AIDS and Adolescents*. Amsterdam: Harwood Academic.

KIPPAX, S., CRAWFORD, J., RODDEN, P. and BENTON, K. (1994) *Report on Project Male-Call: National Telephone Survey of Men Who Have Sex with Men*. Canberra: Australian Government Publishing Service.

McKUSICK, L., COATES, T.J., MORIN, S.F., POLLACK, L. and HOFF, C. (1990) 'Longitudinal predictors of reductions in unprotected anal intercourse among gay men in San Francisco: the AIDS Behavioral Research Project', *American Journal of Public Health*, **80**, pp. 978–83.

MEYER, I.H. and DEAN, L. (1995) 'Patterns of sexual behavior and risk taking among young New York City gay men', *AIDS Education and Prevention*, **7**, suppl., pp. 13–23.

MORRIS, M., ZAVISCA, J. and DEAN, L. (1995) 'Social and sexual networks: their role in the spread of HIV/AIDS among young gay men', *AIDS Education and Prevention*, **7**, suppl., pp. 24–35.

MYERS, T., TUDIVER, F.G., KURTZ, R.G., JACKSON, E.A., ORR, K.W., ROWE, C.J. and BULLOCK, S.L. (1992) 'The Talking Sex Project: descriptions of the study population and correlates of sexual practices at baseline', *Canadian Journal of Public Health*, **83**, pp. 47–52.

RIDGE, D.T., PLUMMER, D.C. and MINICHIELLO, V. (1994) 'Young gay men and HIV: running the risk?', *AIDS Care*, **6**, pp. 371–78.

SCHMIDT, K.W., FOUCHARD, J.R., KRASNIK, A., ZOFFMANN, H., JACOBSEN, H.L. and KREINER, S. (1992) 'Sexual behaviour related to psycho-social factors in a population of Danish homosexual and bisexual men', *Social Science and Medicine*, **34**, pp. 1119–27.

STALL, R., BARRETT, D., BYE, L., CATANIA, J., FRUTCHEY, C., HENNE, J., LEMP, G. and PAUL, J. (1992) 'A comparison of younger and older gay men's HIV risk-taking behaviors: the Communication Technologies 1989 cross-sectional survey', *Journal of Acquired Immune Deficiency Syndromes*, **5**, pp. 682–87.

VALDISERRI, R.O., LYTER, D., LEVITON, L.C., CALLAHAN, C.M., KINGSLEY, L.A. and RINALDO, C.R. (1988) 'Variables influencing condom use in a cohort of gay and bisexual men', *American Journal of Public Health*, **78**, pp. 801–5.

VAN DE VEN, P., KIPPAX, S., CRAWFORD, J., FRENCH, J., PRESTAGE, G., GRULICH, A., KINDER, P. and KALDOR, J. (1997) 'No relationship between age and HIV risk behaviour among Sydney gay men', *AIDS*, **11**, pp. 691–93.

VAN DE VEN, P., NOBLE, J., KIPPAX, S., PRESTAGE, G., CRAWFORD, J., BAXTER, D. and COOPER, D. (1998) 'Gay youth and their precautionary sexual behaviours: the Sydney men and sexual health study', *AIDS Education and Prevention*, **9**, pp. 395–410.

DE WIT, J.B.F. (1996a) 'The epidemic of HIV among young gay men'. Paper presented at the XIth International Conference on AIDS, Vancouver.

DE WIT, J.B.F. (1996b) 'The epidemic of HIV among young homosexual men', *AIDS*, **10**, suppl. 3, pp. 21–25.

DE WIT, J.B.F and VAN GRIENSVEN, G.J.P. (1994) 'Time from safer to unsafe sexual behaviour among homosexual men', *AIDS*, **8**, pp. 123–26.

Chapter 11

A New Method of Peer-Led HIV Prevention with Gay and Bisexual Men

Jonathan Shepherd, Glenn Turner and Katherine Weare

Approaching 20 years into the epidemic, HIV and AIDS continue to affect more gay and bisexual men in England than other groups put together. Figures for 1996 show a record number of HIV infections attributed to sex between men (PHLS, 1997) and studies of sexual behaviour in Britain show that between 1993 and 1995 one-third of gay men surveyed reported episodes of unprotected anal intercourse each year (Hickson *et al.*, 1996). Furthermore, data from the 1997 survey undertaken at the Gay Pride March in London shows no change in the proportions of men reporting unprotected anal intercourse (Hickson, 1997). Explanations for this continuing trend have centred upon evidence that many gay men find it difficult to sustain safer sex practices over time, and periodically engage in episodes of unsafe sex (Ekstrand, 1992; de Wit, *et al.*, 1993). The HIV prevention needs of gay and bisexual men are complex, requiring sophisticated interventions to facilitate risk reduction strategies such as negotiated safety (Davies, *et al.*, 1995; Kippax *et al.*, 1997).

There is also a need to continue to work with those starting their sexual careers to enable them to learn to adopt safer sex as evidence suggests that these, predominantly though not exclusively, younger gay and bisexual men are unlikely to receive HIV prevention education at school which addresses gay sexuality and sexual practices (Frankham, 1995). Therefore, the HIV prevention needs of young gay and bisexual men are variable, depending upon whether they are in the process of adopting or maintaining safer sex (Prochaska, *et al.*, 1994), and contextual, according to the influence of sexual partners (Davies, 1994).

Methods of Preventing HIV: Peer Education

Peer education has been lauded as an effective way to promote safer sex within gay communities (Oakley, Oliver and Peersman, 1995; Kelly *et al.,* 1995; Kippax *et al.*, 1993, Tudiver *et al.*, 1992). Within the gay communities of the UK, North America and Australia peer education has a long-standing history. During the early days of the AIDS epidemic, gay and bisexual men educated each other about safer sex in what has been described as 'informal' peer education (King, 1993; Rooney and Scott, 1991; Scott, 1997). Today peer education initiatives remain a significant part of HIV prevention initiatives within gay communities. Early on in the epidemic, peer education was characterized by its informality and was initiated by gay men themselves in response to an emerging epidemic, but it is now common for peer education initiatives to be initiated, planned and managed by statutory and voluntary health promotion agencies (Deverell, 1995; McKevitt, Warwick and Whitty, 1994).[1] Despite the popularity of peer-led HIV prevention with gay and bisexual men and evidence of its effectiveness (Kelly *et al.*, 1991; Tudiver *et al.*, 1992), there remain a number of issues concerning its efficacy that are in need of clarification.

The Hapeer Project

The HAPEER Project (HIV/AIDS Peer Education Research Project), was a research project set up to investigate the effectiveness of peer education as a method of HIV prevention with young gay and bisexual men. It was based at the Health Education Unit at the University of Southampton and carried out in conjunction with Southampton Gay Men's Health Project (SGMHP). The project conducted an initial needs assessment, recruited and trained a small group of peer educators from the local gay community, and designed and evaluated an intervention in which they participated to promote sexual health.[2] In this chapter we will report briefly upon our evaluation of the process of recruiting and training peer educators, and in greater detail upon the evidence generated by the quasi-experimental evaluation of the intervention in which the peer educators participated. This chapter will therefore focus upon the key learning to arise from the process of implementing the intervention.

The Process of Recruiting and Training Peer Educators

While there is evidence about how volunteers can be recruited to peer education initiatives which have been in existence for some time (Klein, Sondag and Drolet, 1994), it is less clear how a project in its infancy can 'get off the ground' and recruit a core of initial volunteers. The process of training young gay and bisexual men to promote sexual health among their peers is also poorly understood. There is little evidence to guide practitioners to deliver training in a manner which is appropriate to young gay and bisexual men and which ensures their maximum participation in the project, and which adequately prepares them for the role of peer education. It was therefore necessary to evaluate the process of recruitment of peer educators and the training they subsequently received.

During the recruitment stage of the project, the researcher (Jonathan Shepherd) and the project workers from SGMHP (one of them was Glenn Turner) spent a period of three months interacting with young gay and bisexual men within the local gay community, publicizing the project and its impending recruitment. Invitations to introductory project meetings were distributed in the context of one-to-one interactions between the project workers and young gay and bisexual men in gay pubs, clubs and social groups.

Upon recruitment, the peer educators underwent training ($n = 20$) in two groups, one trained by an independent trainer ($n = 10$) and one trained by the two project workers from SGMHP ($n = 10$). The training took place over a 6–8 week period, during one evening a week, based upon a curriculum designed to enable the peer educators to develop the knowledge, skills and abilities to promote sexual health among their peers. Both groups were trained between October and December 1995, and also received additional ongoing training and support throughout the intervention phase of the project. Evaluation of the recruitment and training stages of the project was carried out by the researcher who conducted feedback activities at the end of every training session, and semi-structured interviews with each of the peer educators towards the end of their training programme.

The young gay and bisexual men who participated as peer educators in this project were asked what motivated them to become involved. A variety of reasons were cited, including the perception that it might be an opportunity to meet new people, to acquire new skills and knowledge, and to contribute towards the fight against AIDS. The need for personal growth and altruism are therefore factors which encourage participation in initiatives of this kind, a finding shared by Cassell and Ouellette (1995).

Evaluation of the process of recruitment also found that prior familiarization and interpersonal contact between the project workers, researcher and young gay and bisexual men was a key factor in their initial participation in the project. In particular, familiarization and rapport with project workers during the months preceding the launch of the project stimulated their interest in joining the project and put them at ease during the initial training sessions. Therefore, while initiatives which have been in existence for some time can attract volunteers on the basis of familiarity with the project and observation of its existing peer educators, a new project can recruit a core of new volunteers through the establishment of rapport and familiarity between project workers and potential volunteers.

Evaluation of the training also shed light upon how young gay and bisexual men can be effectively prepared to assume the roles of peer educators. A curriculum was designed to enable them to provide factual information to their peers, facilitate attitude change, teach safer sexual negotiation skills, and facilitate the development of risk reduction strategies with their peers. However, much of the initial training focused upon providing the trainee peer educators with in-depth factual information concerning HIV transmission and prevention. Activities concerning attitudes, safer sexual negotiation skills and risk reduction strategies were therefore postponed for later training sessions. The trainee peer educators' reported that the reason they needed to learn in great detail about the transmission and prevention of HIV and other sexually transmitted diseases was because it provided them with the confidence to assume their roles as peer educators. Many of them considered it important to be able to provide their peers with accurate and up-to-date factual information. They also felt it dangerous to provide information which might not be correct, and upon which their peers might subsequently base their sexual decision making. Although peer educators need to be able to be skilled in a number of activities in order to meet the needs of their peers, a great deal of time needs to be spent enabling them to develop their own knowledge as this provides them with the confidence to begin to develop their sexual health promotion skills and to assume their roles as peer educators.

In terms of training delivery, the informal manner in which the training was conducted, particularly the fact that the training sessions took place in a room set aside in a gay pub where food and drink was available, was a key factor in the peer educators' motivation to attend the training and in their ability to learn. Those who dropped out of the project during the training (who were later interviewed) mentioned that the first couple of training sessions had been too formal, and that this formality was one of the reasons for their departure. All of the peer educators participated in the project during their spare time and considered it to be, among other things, an opportunity to socialize and to enjoy themselves while making a contribution to the promotion of sexual health. The results of this study, and those of others, suggest that informal approaches are a crucial factor in the effectiveness of training and education with young people (Coleman and Ford, 1996; Elliot *et al.*, 1996). Toward the end of their initial training programme, the peer educators began to participate in the main focus of the project – the intervention.

The Peer-Led Intervention

The literature concerning peer-led HIV prevention initiatives within the gay community reveals a number of different activities, or 'interventions', that peer educators have participated in to promote safer sex. For example, studies by Tudiver *et al.* (1992) and Valdiserri *et al.* (1989) found that peer-led group workshops were effective in terms of promoting safer sex. Interventions in which peer educators conduct one-to-one conversations with their peers about safer sex have also proven effective (Kelly *et al.*, 1991). Informal peer-led interventions, such as 'Tupperware' style safer-sex parties held at peer educators homes, have also been evaluated and found to be an effective method in which peer educators can promote safer sex (AIDS Action Committee Safety Net Program, 1989).

Although these studies provide valuable evidence concerning the effectiveness of different methods of peer-led HIV prevention, they were conducted in gay communities which had, at the time, not yet made changes towards the wide-scale adoption of safer sex. They raise a number of questions concerning the ability of peer education to tackle the complexity of young gay and bisexual men's needs. Four key questions were singled out for further investigation.

How can peer educators target people in a range of settings?

It is not clear how peer-led HIV prevention initiatives can target gay and bisexual men in a range of different social and sexual environments, including young men not fully integrated into the gay community. Tudiver *et al.* (1992) found that although peer-led safer-sex workshops were an effective method in which safer sex could be promoted, they tended to attract older, better-educated gay men, rather than younger men and men from ethnic minorities who, they considered, were more inclined to take sexual risks. This raises the question of how to target young gay and bisexual men (or, for that matter, men of any age) not inclined to attend safer-sex workshops. In order to access a range of individuals in a number of settings, an appropriate strategy could be for peer educators to 'seek out' people from within their own sexual and social networks, among whom they can promote safer sex.

How can peer-led interventions be based upon individual HIV prevention needs?

King has highlighted how many HIV prevention campaigns with gay and bisexual men have not been underpinned by any systematic assessment of their needs (King, 1993). Since then a plethora of needs assessments have been conducted, providing a detailed account of the HIV prevention needs of many gay communities in the UK (Scott, 1996). However, although we have a detailed account of community needs, note that needs may vary between individuals, particularly whether they are in the process of adopting or maintaining safer sex. It is not clear how peer educators can identify which issues are appropriate to discuss with each of the individuals they seek to involve in peer education. For example, it would be inappropriate for a peer educator to provide information regarding safer sexual behaviour if an individual already had a sound understanding of HIV transmission and prevention. Consequently, there is a need to investigate how peer educators can assess HIV prevention needs on an individual basis in order to 'start where people are'.

How can peer educators respond to varying needs?

Depending upon the individual needs of each of their peers, peer educators should be equipped to engage in a range of activities such as information provision, teaching sexual negotiation skills, or facilitation of risk reduction strategies development. It is interesting to note that in a study conducted by Valdiserri *et al.* (1989), the most successful component of the intervention concerned the teaching of sexual negotiation skills, yet this component was led by a psychotherapist and did not involve the peer educators at all. The increasing complexity of gay and bisexual men's responses to the epidemic requires equally sophisticated health promotion interventions, and it is clear that we are now asking far more from peer educators than ever before. What is not clear is whether it is realistic to recruit and train peer educators to fully address the agenda for HIV prevention with gay and bisexual men.

How can the effectiveness of peer education interventions
be evaluated?

Peer education has been criticized for failing to provide evidence of its effectiveness (Milburn, 1995). There has been a tendency to evaluate the impact of this method of education solely upon the peer educators themselves rather than among those targeted for peer education (Coleman and Ford, 1996; Wilton *et al.*, 1995). Recent calls for greater rigour in the evaluation of sexual health promotion interventions, including the assessment of outcome measures such as changes in knowledge, attitudes and behaviour over time, highlight the importance of establishing effective and practical ways in which peer-led interventions can be evaluated (Bonell, 1996; Oakley *et al.*, 1995). However, there are difficulties inherent in evaluating the effectiveness of peer education, especially interventions such as peer-led one-to-one interactions which take place in informal settings. For example, although peer educators may have access to individuals within their social and sexual networks to provide information, support and advice in the form of informal discussions and conversations, an evaluator may not have the same access to such networks in order to assess what impact peer education has had upon those involved. Consequently, there is a need to identify practical and realistic methods of evaluating the impact of informal peer-led interventions upon those targeted, in terms of outcome measures such as knowledge, attitudes and behaviour, over time.

How the intervention was devised

The intervention was therefore devised and evaluated in order to clarify these four key research questions. It was designed as an 'outreach' method to

Table 11.1 Specification of the Intervention

Each peer educator conducts a *structured interview* with around five individuals that they come into contact with in the gay community. During the interview they ask questions about
• their knowledge of HIV/AIDS and sexually transmitted diseases
• their attitudes towards sexual health and sexual lifestyles
• their use of local sexual health services
• their sexual behaviour

The *purpose* of the interview is to
• provide the peer educator with an indication of the needs of the individual
• provide a springboard for a discussion on sexual health
• provide baseline data for evaluation of the intervention

Having conducted the interview, the peer educator may then respond to the identified needs through *discussion*.

After the interview the peer educator responds to their *ongoing needs* as and when required by the individual and/or when the peer educator considers it to be appropriate.

The interview is then repeated at a *follow-up period* of three months.

The *purpose* of this follow-up interview is to
• allow the peer educator to further identify and respond to the sexual health needs of the individual
• provide post-intervention data for the evaluation of the intervention

---

overcome the problem of low attendance at workshop-style interventions, an issue we mentioned earlier (Table 11.1). The task for the peer educators was to seek out a small sample of individuals with whom they regularly interacted, typically whomever they felt comfortable with, with whom they would conduct short structured interviews on the topic of sexual health. A structured interview was considered to be easier for the peer educators to conduct than an unstructured interview. A structured interview requires the interviewer to ask the questions exactly as they are worded on the schedule and to tick or write in the responses in the relevant boxes. An unstructured interview requires the interviewer to adopt a more flexible approach, prompting and probing according to the responses of the interviewer (Cohen and Manion, 1994). Although both require the interviewer to be trained, an unstructured interview requires considerably more skill to conduct than a structured interview (Oppenheim, 1993).

It was intended that upon completion of the interview, a conversation would ensue in which the interviewee would have the opportunity to ask any questions relating to their sexual health needs, and in which the peer educator could respond to any needs that they considered to be relevant, as identified by the interview. The data generated from the interview would not only enable the peer educators to assess 'where people are', but would also be used as a baseline from which changes in knowledge, attitudes and behaviour could be assessed, therefore enabling outcomes to be measured. The interview therefore fulfilled three roles – a vehicle for initiation of discussion, a method of ascertaining individual needs and a tool for evaluation.

Each peer educator was requested to respond to the needs of their targeted peers on an ongoing basis, typically over a period of three to six months, whenever they felt it was appropriate, or whenever their peers required their assistance. Upon completion of this interim period, the peer educators could then re-interview their peers, using the same interview schedule, to ascertain whether any changes had occurred in their knowledge, attitudes and behaviour.

The intervention took place between January and August 1996, during which time the 11 remaining peer educators targeted a total of 43 gay and bisexual men. The lowest number of people targeted per peer educator was 2, the highest was 7, with an average of around 4. A comparison group was included in the study; they did not receive the intervention but they were interviewed by the researcher at baseline then between three and six months later. Individuals in this group were sampled in a neighbouring gay community to lessen the chances of them coming into contact with the peer educators in the intervention community.

Evaluation of the Intervention

The evaluation sought to establish whether the intervention was effective in meeting its predefined objectives of changing, where appropriate, knowledge, attitudes and behaviour, and to clarify the four key research questions outlined earlier.

What impact did the intervention have upon those targeted?

In terms of outcomes, at baseline both the intervention group and those in the comparison group generally had an accurate knowledge of HIV/AIDS transmission and prevention; a basic understanding of sexually transmitted diseases; relatively tolerant attitudes towards gay and bisexual lifestyles; and reported low levels of unsafe sex. At follow-up in the intervention group there was a slight increase in knowledge of HIV/AIDS transmission and prevention and a statistically significant increase in knowledge of the prevention and transmission of other sexually transmitted diseases, relative to the comparison group. Very little change in attitudes and reported sexual behaviour were observed in both the intervention and comparison groups. Data is presented for these outcomes in Shepherd, Weare and Turner (1997).

How did the peer educators negotiate interviews with their peers?

The peer educators employed a variety of methods to negotiate interviews with their peers. In terms of finding people to interview, their strategies ranged from the opportunistic to the carefully targeted. Some took the opportunity to ask friends who happened to be visiting their homes if they would like to be interviewed, whereas others took a more proactive approach, typically making an intentional visit to a friend's house to interview them. For example, one peer educator, together with his flatmate, reported that he regularly cooked breakfast for a group of their friends every Sunday morning, during which time he took the opportunity to interview some of them. In contrast, another peer educator, who was a member of a local gay youth group, took his interview folder with him on a number of occasions with the intention of interviewing people while at the group.

There was also variation in the techniques employed to negotiate interviews. Some peer educators simply asked their peers if they would like to be interviewed, whereas others devised strategies to advertise and promote the interview. For example, one peer educator claimed that he employed what he described as 'marketing' techniques to promote the interview to his friends. He deliberately made it sound desirable to stimulate their interest, and he found this was an effective strategy. In nearly all cases the peer educators encountered little resistance when negotiating the interviews; none encountered a refusal.

How were the interviews conducted?

The peer educators employed a variety of techniques and methods to conduct their interviews. The majority of the interviews involved the peer educators asking the questions on the interview schedule and afterwards discussing sexual health with their peers, although some of the peer educators tailored the interview to suit their preferred methods and techniques. For example, some of them asked the questions first and left the conversation until afterwards (as recommended by the researcher), whereas others preferred to discuss particular issues as they arose during the interview, primarily because it facilitated the flow of the conversation. As one peer educator remarked:

> Trying to save answering their questions till later didn't work, trying to go back to talking about it at the end didn't work so well as talking about it there and then, because it made it flow so much better.

Similarly, another peer educator preferred to discuss issues as they arose during the interview, taking care not to influence the interviewees' answers to subsequent questions:

> We went through the questions and I used them in that order . . . if they wanted to talk about it there and then I would move the conversation round to the next question and then have another discussion about that.

None of the peer educators reported any significant problems associated with their ability to elicit information from their interviewees.

There was also evidence to suggest that the interview was an effective method of stimulating discussion on the subject of HIV and sexual health. In the majority of cases the interviews took around 5 to 10 minutes to complete whereas the ensuing conversations varied in duration from 5 minutes to 2 hours, to a whole evening, depending upon the needs of the interviewee. The average duration of the discussions was around 20 minutes. Many of the longer conversations were not exclusively concerned with sexual health. Some of the peer educators reported that on many occasions the conversation progressed onto issues concerning love and relationships, and sometimes digressed into more general gossip! Yet, periodically these conversations would return to issues relating to sexual health either by chance or through the guidance of the peer educator.

The interviews generally proceeded without any problems and were considered by the peer educators to be an enjoyable experience. Mostly this was because those interviewed were their close friends and associates, and it was an opportunity for them to have a chat and a laugh. Indeed, some sought to strike a balance in approach between the serious and the light-hearted. In the majority of cases the peer educators enjoyed their interviews and felt that their peers enjoyed it too. The majority of the discussions involved the active participation of the interviewees in the conversation.

What happened during the interim period?

During the interval, or 'interim period', between the initial and follow-up interviews the majority of the peer educators made it known to their peers that they were available at any time if they ever needed support and information. One peer educator reported that his interviewees had approached him on several occasions to ask him further questions relating to HIV/AIDS and sexually transmitted diseases:

> One of these people I actually live with and on a regular basis we still talk about safer sex . . . it is an ongoing saga . . . it is just routine now because obviously I see these people regularly and we chat.

Another peer educator commented that, through his involvement in the project, people perceived him to be a point of reference for matters relating to sexual health and sex in general:

> It is like being part of tourist information isn't it, I get loads of e-mails at work saying, 'Where are good trolling places?' . . . You become like the good trolling guide!

Nevertheless, the majority of the peer educators reported that, despite regular contact during the interim period with the peers they had interviewed, sexual health was rarely discussed. Some of them suggested that it was only through conducting the follow-up interview that sexual health matters were talked about further. Some of them regarded the follow-up interview, rather than being an end in itself, as the second stage of a process of dialogue concerning sexual health:

> I think it takes longer than just two sessions to really get it to sink in, not in all cases but generally speaking I think most of them appreciate the chance to continue . . . it is only a start really.

One of the peer educators remarked that, although the interview was a good method of initiating discussion about sexual health, there was a need for another method of sparking off conversation during the interim period between interviews:

> I wouldn't say to do an interview every time you see them, but I think its important to be able to use the interviews to set up an environment where you can talk to them again about it without having to get out an interview sheet. . . . I still think that once every three months may not really be enough to get a message across.

Therefore, although there was evidence of some ongoing peer education during the interim period, it was generally the case that sexual health was rarely discussed.

What were the skills and abilities of the peer educators?

In terms of competencies, information provision was the activity in which the majority of the peer educators considered themselves to be most effective. Nearly all the interviews focused, to a great extent, upon the provision of information about HIV and sexual health, and increases in knowledge among those targeted for peer education were observed:

> I found knowledge quite easy to do because it is ... education is
> supposed to be about facts.

Some of the peer educators therefore had a conception of education as
primarily concerned with information giving. Many of them commented that
they were comfortable providing factual information because it was more
straightforward than discussing attitudes which as one person described, had
more 'grey areas'.

Among those targeted for peer education, attitudes towards safer sex and
sexual lifestyles were generally tolerant and there was little change in attitudes
over time. Although peer educators recognized that the objective was to
increase tolerance to sexual lifestyles, some of them did not feel comfortable
trying to change people's attitudes, and avoided discussing them:

> I particularly didn't like trying to change people's attitudes. People's
> attitudes are grounded in long-standing opinions and they may
> change over time but I am not really sure it's my job to do that.

Others avoided addressing them for other reasons. For example, they felt that
many of the attitudinal issues were too complex and they did not want to go
into great detail. In contrast, a couple of the peer educators found discussing
attitudes to be an interesting experience:

> I am interested in like you know the sort of sociology of it you know
> what makes people tick ... you think you know someone quite well
> and they can really surprise you with some of their opinions.

Those who did address attitudes felt that they had limited success in
achieving any form of measurable change. They recognized that attitude
change is a lengthy process and that the most they could do was to raise
awareness of some of the relevant issues; as one person put it, 'to get the ball
rolling'.

The practices of safer and unsafe sex were not talked about in great depth
during the interviews for a number of reasons. The majority of those targeted
were, at the time, practising safer sex and the peer educators did not always
consider discussion of safer sex to be necessary. In these cases, rather than
taking a proactive role and discussing future potential episodes of unprotected
anal intercourse, the peer educators took a passive approach, offering to be on
hand whenever needed for any advice or support their peers might require to
continue having safer sex.

There were some instances in which discussion of sexual behaviour was
relevant, primarily in cases where the interviewee reported a recent episode of
unsafe sex. For example, one peer educator reported that he and his interviewee reflected upon a particular unsafe encounter and together identified
ways in which this could be prevented from happening in the future:

It was basically going through the scenario that happened and looking at the opportunities that they could have used to have a condom
to hand.

In this case the peer educator was attempting to facilitate the development of
skills to negotiate safer sex.

There were also instances in which the peer educator considered that
discussion of the unsafe encounter was not appropriate. In one case, an
interviewee was aware of why he had unsafe sex and did not rule out the
possibility that it might happen again. In this situation the peer educator
reported that he did not pursue this and was very conscious of the fact that
his intervention on this matter could be interpreted as 'preaching'. All of
the peer educators asserted that they did not want to apply any form of
peer pressure for a number of reasons. Specifically, it was considered that
it would be counterproductive and would not have any impact upon then
interviewees' behaviour. Rather, the peer educators considered that their
role was to inform their peers of the risks associated with unprotected anal
intercourse.

The few occasions when the peer educators discussed risk reduction
strategies with their peers did not always proceed without problems. For
example, one peer educator elaborated upon an occasion in which he
discussed negotiated safety with one of his interviewees. The interviewee and
his regular partner were considering abandoning the use of condoms with
each other on the basis of knowledge of each other's HIV status. The peer
educator was attempting to introduce the issue of trust to the conversation,
specifically, whether the interviewee was sure that he could trust his partner
not to have unprotected anal intercourse with other partners, thus increasing
the likelihood of introducing HIV into the relationship. In short, he was
attempting to ensure that this particular negotiation of safety involved as
few risks as possible. Yet, even though he knew the interviewee as a close
friend, he was unable to bring up the issue of trust in case he took offence,
thinking that he was implying that his partner was being unfaithful. He felt
that this would have negative implications for his friendship with the
interviewee:

> I think it might have fucked up the whole of the rest of the interview
> really and it would have made me appear to be taking sides almost,
> and I think he would be a bit reluctant to confide in me in the future,
> which I don't want to risk.

In this case, although familiarity between the peer educator and the interviewee limited the discussion of particular sexual issues, it is possible that with
greater experience and skill he may have been able to tackle the issue without
threatening their friendship.

Discussion

Evaluation of this intervention highlighted the strengths and limitations of this particular method of peer education, and indeed peer education in general, in terms of its abilities to meet the variable and complex HIV prevention needs of young gay and bisexual men.

Targeting Individuals in a Range of Settings

This research was able to identify some of the merits associated with the outreach nature of this intervention. Through encouraging the peer educators to 'seek out' individuals from within their sexual and social networks, they were able to target friends and associates within the context of their day-to-day lives at times and places that were convenient for both parties. One of the advantages of this intervention is that those targeted are not required to assume a proactive role to receive peer education. For example, they do not have to attend events such as safer-sex training workshops, which in the study by Tudiver *et al.* (1992) suffered low attendance from younger men, men from minority ethnic groups, and less well-educated men. Rather, in this intervention the peer educators take on the responsibility of identifying individuals from within their personal networks to target for peer education. The evidence from our research suggests that this was a task the peer educators achieved with few problems.

Although the majority of men targeted had regular contact with the gay commercial scene, in which there was existing provision of sexual health information and advice, the outreach nature of the intervention enabled the peer educators to target a proportion of individuals either not integrated into the gay community or whose contact with the community was infrequent. Our earlier research and the work of others shows that these individuals do not always have access to the 'gay-specific' information, advice and support provided in gay environments (Kippax *et al.*, 1993; Shepherd, 1995).

Assessing Individual Needs

The data generated by the interviews provided the peer educators with a profile of the needs of each of their interviewees. Through asking the questions specified on the interview schedule, they were able to 'start where people are' by focusing their education and support, to the best of their abilities, upon the most appropriate issues. The length of the ensuing discussions often varied according to the needs of the individuals resulting in, where appropriate, in-depth discussion concerning factual information and in some cases attitudes and sexual behaviour.

Responding to Varying Needs

In order to fully address the agenda for HIV prevention, peer education – like any other form of education – needs to be able to provide information, facilitate attitude change, teach sexual negotiation skills and to address the complexities of risk reduction strategies. The results of our research suggest that, generally, the peer educators were more comfortable and effective in their role as information providers than agents of attitude and behaviour change. They underwent training to prepare them for their role, based upon a curriculum designed to enable them to develop the knowledge and skills to promote sexual health. However, much of the training programme was devoted to meeting their need to develop in-depth knowledge regarding HIV/AIDS and other sexually transmitted diseases, primarily because knowledge acquisition boosted their confidence, a necessary prerequisite to begin working as peer educators. Although they received ongoing training to enable them to further develop their abilities, it was generally the case that during the short timescale of the project they were more comfortable and effective at providing information. It is possible that if the project had continued for another year, the peer educators may have further developed their abilities to discuss risk reduction strategies or teach safer sexual negotiation skills. Further research is needed into ways in which health promotion specialists can train peer educators to tackle complex sexual issues.

Evaluating Outcomes

The interview fulfilled its purpose as an evaluative tool. The data derived from the initial interviews was used to set a baseline of the knowledge, attitudes and behaviour of every person targeted, a baseline against which the effectiveness of peer education could be measured. The data elicited during the follow-up interviews enabled the measurement of changes in outcomes to be achieved. The fact that the majority of those interviewed were close friends of the peer educators with whom they had regular communication, enabled the peer educators to contact them over time to conduct the follow-up interview with relative ease, lessening the problem of attrition, or 'drop-out', commonly experienced in evaluative studies of this kind. Out of the 43 targeted for peer education 35 were followed up, a drop-out of only 8.

It is possible that there was a potential for conflict for the peer educators between their roles as educators and evaluators. It could be the case that those targeted by the peer educators might be inclined to report more favourable changes in knowledge, attitudes and behaviour during the follow-up interview in order to create the impression that the advice, information or teaching provided to them by the peer educator had been effective, rather than offend them in any way by suggesting that it was not adequate. While it is not possible to determine whether those targeted for the intervention had overstated the effectiveness of the intervention they received, the peer educators in this study did not report any conflict in their combined role as educators and evaluators, and they commented that those they had targeted had no obvious reason to report false answers.

Furthermore, it is unlikely that the peer educators felt pressured in any way to be effective. Although they were aware that the interviews they were conducting provided evaluation data, the main purpose of the interviews was as a tool for education. Their perception of their role was primarily to educate rather than evaluate. They merely collected the evaluation data, which was then passed on to the researcher for analysis. The peer educators and their targeted peers were aware that they were taking part in a piece of research in which favourable outcomes were desirable but not essential, as the aim of the investigation was to ascertain the advantages and disadvantages of peer education in preventing HIV. Therefore, it is unlikely that those targeted were inclined to overstate the impact the intervention had upon them, and it is also unlikely that the peer educators felt pressured to achieve a high standard of performance.

The Way Forward

For those interested in implementing this type of intervention, we suggest a number of ways forward to enhance its effectiveness. One method to reduce the time required for training peer educators is to recruit and select peer educators who are already in command of 'general' skills and attributes necessary for education and training (e.g. communication skills or the ability to preserve confidentiality). However, such individuals may still need to learn to apply their skills within the context of peer-led HIV prevention, which may require considerable time and confidence building. It is therefore important to allow time for their development when planning initiatives. The greatest achievement of the peer educators in this project during the year in which they participated was the provision of factual information concerning HIV and other sexually transmitted diseases. It is possible that having proceeded for a longer time they may have begun to develop their abilities to teach sexual negotiation skills or address risk reduction strategies. It is therefore recommended that initiatives are planned with considerable time for peer educators' development in mind.

During the first six to twelve months of participation, the peer educators may be most effective in terms of their ability to provide factual information. Therefore it may be appropriate during the first year of a peer-led HIV prevention initiative to encourage them to target individuals who have a need for basic factual information regarding HIV transmission and prevention. These individuals are likely to be younger gay and bisexual men making their sexual debut, some of whom will be in the process of becoming integrated into the mainstream gay community. To achieve this it will be necessary to recruit peer educators whose sexual and social networks extend beyond the main-stream gay community, so they can target those who may not be integrated into established spheres of gay sexual and social activity. Over time, with ongoing training and support, the peer educators may gradually start to feel confident enough to begin targeting individuals whose needs may be more complex, people with whom they may, where appropriate, facilitate the development of sexual negotiation skills, attitude change or risk reduction strategies.

This intervention could be interpreted as an 'intensive' method of peer education which can be employed to complement other 'extensive' initiatives within a gay community. At 43 the number of gay and bisexual men targeted for peer education in this project was relatively low, especially when the average number of people targeted by each peer educator was 4. However, the average length of each discussion was 20 minutes, and some lasted 2 hours or more. Therefore, the value of this intervention lies in its ability to address HIV, and where necessary other sexual health issues, and to address them in depth, something which has been proposed as an appropriate method for addressing the complex sexual strategies employed by many gay and bisexual men. The intervention took place in a gay community in which a range of sexual health initiatives ran concurrently, provided by Southampton Gay Men's Health Project. Many of these initiatives were designed to reach a larger audience, such as outreach activities in pubs and clubs catering for large gatherings of people, but perhaps not in such depth as this particular interven-tion. Therefore, this intervention could be implemented in other, similar communities as a way of complementing existing 'extensive' initiatives.

Conclusion

The fight against AIDS has been fraught with many difficulties as well as some remarkable successes. We have good evidence of the effectiveness of health promotion initiatives to prevent HIV transmission, yet there remain many unanswered questions and there is much to learn. This study was conducted at a time when, despite considerable behaviour changes made by gay men to safer sex in the 1980s, we are confronted by recent surveys showing around one-third of gay and bisexual men reporting episodes of unsafe sex each year, coupled with an all-time high of HIV infections attributed to sex between men during 1996 in the UK. The agenda for HIV prevention with gay and bisexual men is to enable them to maintain safer sexual practices – an increasingly sophisticated and complex task – and to encourage the adoption of safer sex among those making their sexual debut. Despite evidence of the effectiveness of peer education within gay communities, there is a lack of knowledge regard-ing specific effective methods of peer education. There is even less evidence of the effectiveness of peer education, or for that matter health education in general, at tackling the complex emerging strategies employed by many gay men during the second decade of the epidemic. This study has endeavoured to address this paucity of knowledge.

The agenda for HIV prevention towards the close of the twentieth century is more challenging, requiring careful targeting, assessment of individual needs and multiple educational strategies and techniques. The key question we have addressed is: To what extent can peer education take on this more complex and varied agenda? Approaching 20 years into the epidemic, we are asking a great deal more of peer educators in terms of knowledge, skills and flexibility of response. We have designed and evaluated an intervention and found it to be flexible and adaptable, and one which facilitates, where appropriate and to the best of the peer educators' abilities, in-depth discussion concerning the feelings, meanings and constructs associated with safer sex. Our evidence suggests that peer educators need support over a lengthy period of time and that the process needs to be highly structured, although not necessarily too formal.

It is important to acknowledge that gay and bisexual men continue to play an important role in educating, informing and supporting one another in the fight against AIDS. The challenge for future research is to investigate how they can be supported to contribute to an effective health promotion response to a continuing and changing epidemic.

Acknowledgements

Thanks go to all of the peer educators who took part in the project; their input was crucial to this research. We are grateful to (the former) Wessex Regional Health Authority Research and Development Taskforce (HIV/AIDS and Sexual Health) for funding this research. Thanks also go to Southampton Gay Men's Health Project, particularly to Neil Dacombe for all his help.

Notes

1 An exception is the voluntary organization Gay Men Fighting AIDS (GMFA) which promotes peer education as a practice and a philosophy, and is initiated and planned by gay men themselves.
2 The scope of the project was limited primarily to HIV prevention. However, the results of the first stage of the project, a needs assessment (Shepherd, 1995), recommended widening the scope to include the prevention of other sexually transmitted diseases. The peer educators promoted aspects of sexual health such as the prevention of hepatitis B, gonorrhoea and testicular cancer during their involvement with the project as well as HIV; however, this chapter takes HIV and AIDS as its main focus, specifically the ability of peer education to meet the agenda for HIV prevention.

References

AIDS ACTION COMMITTEE SAFETY NET PROGRAM (1989) 'Notes from the field: small group parties for safer sex education', *American Journal of Public Health*, **79**, pp. 1305–6.

BONELL, C. (1996) *Outcomes in HIV Prevention – Report of a Research Project*. London: HIV Project.

CASSEL, J.B. and OUELLETTE, S. (1995) 'A typology of AIDS volunteers', *AIDS Education and Prevention*, **7**, suppl. pp. 80–90.

COHEN, L. and MANION, L. (1994) *Research Methods in Education*. London Routledge.

COLEMAN, L.M. and FORD, N.J. (1996) 'An extensive literature review of the evaluation of HIV prevention programmes', *Health Education Research: Theory and Practice*, **11**, pp. 327–38.

DAVIES, P.M. (1994) 'Acts, sessions and individuals: a model for analysing sexual behaviour', in Boulton, M. (ed.) *Challenge and Innovation: Methodological Advances in Social Research on HIV/AIDS*. London: Taylor & Francis.

DAVIES, P. M., HICKSON, F., BEARDSELL, S. and WEATHERBURN, P. (1995) The maintenance of safer sexual behaviour among gay and bisexual men in the UK: a report to the Health Education Authority. Unpublished draft report, SIGMA Research, London.

DEVERELL, K. (1995) *KY Babies Peer Education Project – Evaluation Final Report*. London: HIV Project.

EKSTRAND, M.L. (1992) 'Safer sex maintenance among gay men: are we making any progress?', *AIDS*, **6**, pp. 875–77.

ELLIOTT, L., GRUER, L., FARROW, K., HENDERSON, A. and COWAN, L. (1996) 'Theatre in AIDS education – a controlled study', *AIDS Care*, **8**, 3, pp. 321–40.

FRANKHAM, J. (1995) *Young Gay Men and HIV Infection*. Horsham: AVERT.

HICKSON, F. (1997) 'Treatment advances and risk taking', *CHAPS*, No. 3, Nov/Dec.

HICKSON, F.C.I., REID, D.S., DAVIES, P.M., WEATHERBURN, P., BEARDSELL, S. and KEOGH, P.G. (1996) 'No aggregate change in homosexual HIV risk behaviour among gay men attending the gay pride festivals, United Kingdom, 1993–1995', *AIDS*, **10**, pp. 771–74.

KELLY, J. (1995) *Changing HIV Risk Behaviour: Practical Strategies*. New York: Guildford Press.

KELLY, J.A., ST LAWRENCE, J.S., STEVENSON, Y.L., HAUTH, A.C., KALICHMAN, S.C., DIAZ, Y.E., BRASFIELD, T.L., KOOB, J.J. and MORGAN, M.G. (1991) 'Featuring HIV/AIDS: community AIDS/HIV risk reduction – the effects of endorsements by popular people in three cities', *American Journal of Public Health*, **81**, pp. 168–71

KING, E. (1993) *Safety in Numbers*. London: Cassell.

KIPPAX, S., CONNELL, R., DOWSETT, G. and CRAWFORD, J. (1993) *Sus-*

taining Safer Sex: Gay Communities Respond to AIDS. London: Falmer Press.

KIPPAX, S., NOBLE, J., PRESTAGE, G., CRAWFORD, J., CAMPBELL, D., BAXTER, D. and COOPER, D. (1997) 'Sexual negotiation in the AIDS era: negotiated safety revisited', *AIDS*, **11**, pp. 191–97.

KLEIN, N.A., SONDAG, K.A. and DROLET, J.C. (1994) 'Understanding volunteer peer health educators' motivations: applying social learning theory', *Journal of American College Health*, **43**, p. 126.

McKEVITT, C., WARWICK, I. and WHITTY, G. (1994) *Health First Peer Education Project – Evaluation Final Report*. London: Health First/Health and Education Research Unit, Institute of Education, University of London.

MILBURN, K. (1995) 'A critical review of peer education with young people with special reference to sexual health', *Health Education Research: Theory and Practice*, **10**, p. 407.

OAKLEY, A., OLIVER, S. and PEERSMAN, G. (1995) *Review of the Effectiveness of Health Promotion Interventions for Men Who Have Sex with Men*. London: Epi Centre, Social Science Research Unit, Institute of Education, University of London.

OAKLEY, A., FULLERTON, D., HOLLAND, J., ARNOLD, S., FRANCE-DAWSON, M., KELLEY, P. and McGRELLIS, S. (1995) 'Sexual health education interventions for young people: a methodological review', *British Medical Journal*, **310**, pp. 158–62.

OPPENHEIM, A.N. (1993) *Questionnaire Design, Interviewing and Attitude Measurement*. London: Pinters.

PHLS AIDS CENTRE, COMMUNICABLE DISEASE SURVEILLANCE CENTRE AND SCOTTISH CENTRE FOR INFECTION AND ENVIRONMENTAL HEALTH (1997) Unpublished Quarterly Surveillance Tables No. 34, Data to end December 1996.

PROCHASKA, J.O., REDDING, C.A., HARLOW, L.L., ROSSI, J.S. and VELICER, W.F. (1994) 'The transtheoretical model of change and HIV prevention: a review', *Health Education Quarterly*, **21**, p. 471.

ROONEY, M. and SCOTT, P. (1991) 'Working where the risks are', in Evans, B., Sandberg, S. and Watson, I. (eds) *Working Where the Risks Are*. London: Health Education Authority.

SCOTT, P. (1996) *Moving Targets: An Assessment of the Needs of Gay Men and Bisexual Men in Relation to HIV Prevention in Enfield and Haringey*. London: Enfield and Haringey Health Authority.

SCOTT, P. (1997) 'How gay men's activism gets written out of AIDS prevention', in Oppenheimer, J. and Beckitt, H. (eds) *Acting on AIDS: Sex, Drugs and Politics*. London: Serpent's Tail.

SHEPHERD, J. (1995) *An investigation into effective HIV prevention with young gay and bisexual men – the HAPEER project*. Interim Report, May 1995. Southampton: University of Southampton Health Education Unit, School of Education.

SHEPHERD, J., WEARE, K. and TURNER, G. (1997) 'Peer-led sexual health promotion with young gay and bisexual men – results of the HAPEER project, *Health Education*, **6**, 204–12.

TUDIVER, R., MYERS, T., KURTZ, R.G., ORR, K., ROWE, C., JACKSON, E. and BULLOCK, S.L. (1992) 'The talking sex project: results of a randomized controlled trial of small group AIDS education for 612 gay and bisexual men', *Evaluation and the Health Professions*, **15**, pp. 26–42

VALDISERRI, R.O., LYTER, D.W., LEVITON, L.C., CALLAHAN, C.M., KINGSLEY, L.A. and RINALDO, C.R. (1989) 'AIDS prevention in homosexual and bisexual men: results of a randomized trial evaluating two risk reduction interventions', *AIDS*, **1**, pp. 21–26.

WILTON, T., KEEBLE, S., DOYAL, L. and WALSH, A. (1995) *The Effectiveness of Peer Education in Health Promotion: Theory and Practice*. Report to the South and West Research and Development Directorate, University of the West of England, Faculty of Health and Community Studies.

DE WIT, J., GRIENSVEN, G. VAN, KOK, G. and SANDFORT, T. (1993) 'Why do homosexual men relapse into unsafe sex? Predictors of resumption of unprotected anogenital intercourse with casual partners', *AIDS*, **7**, pp. 1113–18.

Chapter 12

Sexual Risk Taking and HIV Testing: A Qualitative Investigation

Susan Beardsell

Whether or not HIV testing should be more widely promoted has been an issue of some controversy from the beginning of the epidemic, and one which is likely to intensify given recent developments in drug therapies. Apart from treatment benefits, however, 'pro-testing' positions have suggested that testing can have a public health benefit by facilitating behaviour change to prevent the transmission of HIV and many commentators have seen risk reduction as an important component of the testing process (Beardsell, 1994). There have been numerous research studies which have investigated the relationship between testing and behaviour change. Past reviews (Higgins *et al.*, 1991; Beardsell, 1994) and more recent research (e.g. Allen *et al.*, 1993; Pickering *et al.*, 1993; Desenclos *et al.*, 1993; Delgado-Rodriguez *et al.*, 1994; Kelly, Murphy and Bahr, 1993; Doll and Kennedy, 1994; Ickovics *et al.*, 1994; des Jarlais *et al.*, 1995; Roffman *et al.*, 1995; Wolitski *et al.*, 1997), however, indicate that current evidence is contradictory. Given these findings, and the methodological limitations of much research (Beardsell, 1994), the supposed public health benefit of testing is open to question. The vast majority of studies, moreover, have concentrated on examining the outcomes of testing – whether behaviour change does or does not occur – using highly structured quantitative research methodologies (Beardsell and Coyle, 1996). They thus provide little insight into the mechanisms of behaviour change (or lack thereof) or the relative contribution of testing compared to other factors. This chapter presents a study which aimed to rectify this. It investigated the relationship between HIV testing and behaviour change using a qualitative methodology, focusing on the process of behaviour change – not *if* it occurs but *why* it does or does not take place.

Methods

The sample consisted of 40 women and 51 men who had tested for HIV in the two years prior to interview (Table 12.1). This data is drawn from a larger qualitative research study entitled Service and Psychosocial Issues in HIV Testing funded by the Department of Health and the former North Thames

Table 12.1   Sample for investigating sexual risk taking

	HIV+	HIV−
Women[a]	13	27
Straight men	7	16
Gay/bisexual men	15	13

Age range = 18–47
17 (19%) were members of Black or minority ethnic
  communities
9 (10%) were sex workers
29 (32%) were current or ex-injecting drug users
54 (59%) had taken an HIV test before

[a] Two women were lesbians, one HIV+ and one HIV−.

(East) Regional Health Authority. Following Strauss and Corbin (1990), theoretical sampling was adopted to ensure a full range of differences on dimensions of interest (sex, sexuality, HIV status, history of drug use, past testing experience, type of testing site, etc.). Our aim was to include as diverse a range of experiences and opinions as possible, rather than obtain a 'representative' sample.

Respondents were recruited from a range of sources: (1) via HIV testing sites and statutory and voluntary services for people with HIV in London and the home counties; (2) via advertisements in the gay press, in local newspapers, in magazines (such as *Time Out*, the *Big Issue* and *Miss London*) and in the Body Positive and Mainliners newsletters; and (3) via snowballing. For recruiting via services, appropriate Ethics Committee approval was obtained. While the majority of respondents had their last test in London or the home counties, they also reported on past testing experiences elsewhere in the UK or abroad.

Respondents took part in interviews which lasted from 45 minutes to over 2 hours. The interviews consisted of open-ended questions and respondents were encouraged to discuss issues in depth. Interviews were conducted primarily by the author although all potential respondents were given the option of a male interviewer. Interviews were tape-recorded and full transcripts made. Transcripts were analyzed by two researchers using a grounded theory approach (Glaser and Strauss, 1967) to identify recurrent themes. Analysis focused on identifying themes common to a number of respondents and not on identifying differences on the basis of epidemiological or sociodemographic characteristics. However, when themes were associated predominantly with a particular group of respondents (those with HIV, gay men, sex workers, etc.) this will be reported. This analysis focuses on penetrative vaginal and anal intercourse because only a minority of respondents conceptualized oral sex as posing a significant risk for HIV.

The Role of Counselling in Behaviour Change

Any discussion of HIV testing and behaviour change should account for both the effects of the test and pre- and post-test counselling or discussion. However, the content and methods of test counselling vary enormously and range from a few minutes with a doctor to an hour with a professional counsellor (Beardsell, Hickson and Weatherburn, 1995). Respondents reported that while service providers invariably mentioned safer sex, this often consisted of simply explaining what safer sex is or just advising them 'to be safe', although, the vast majority had very good knowledge of the mechanics of safer sex. Very few service providers helped clients to develop personal risk reduction strategies, and only a tiny minority of respondents believed that discussions with service providers during test sessions had any impact on their attitudes or behaviour.

The Relationship between Risk and Testing

Although past quantitative research has often assumed there is a linear relationship between risk behaviours and testing (Beardsell, 1994), we found the situation to be more complex. The baseline for any behaviour change was not uniform, because the level or extent of 'risk' deemed necessary to warrant a test varied enormously. For example, some respondents believed that 'it only takes once' for infection to occur and tested following a single incident of unprotected intercourse. But more often risk is cumulative, and unprotected intercourse is only deemed risky enough to test once it has occurred a critical number of times, or with a critical number of different partners. This critical number is arbitrary and varies across individuals. Some respondents believed that 'just the once won't hurt' and associated little or no risk with isolated incidents.

> I didn't think I was really at risk. I think there's only really a couple of times I've ever really had anal sex . . . I don't really sort of have anal sex with my partner because I don't really like it very much and I could only think of . . . maybe once on holiday in Spain and once in the Canaries. I could really only think of, you know, two instances in all that time. (Gay man, HIV+)

Assessing personal risk for HIV was not therefore simply a function of engaging in a certain behaviour and testing was not an immediate response to risk. Some HIV positive respondents had not perceived themselves to be at risk at all and sometimes it was only the presence of additional cues, like symptoms or the diagnosis of a partner, ex-partner or baby, that led them (or others) to suspect they might be seropositive. This accords with other evidence that suggests some HIV-infected people do not believe themselves to be infected, even if they acknowledge risk factors (e.g., Zapka *et al.*, 1991; Beevor and Catalan, 1993; Wenger *et al.*, 1994).

The Relationship between Testing and Behaviour Change

Some 60 per cent of HIV negative and 25 per cent of HIV positive respondents reported unprotected intercourse in the period between testing and interview. This data, however, masks a complex hierarchy of behaviour from one-off incidents to multiple incidents with multiple partners, and with different levels of concern as to the perceived riskiness of these behaviours.

When considering whether testing 'works' in terms of behaviour change, quantitative researchers have considered two behavioural patterns before and after testing. Firstly, the respondent engages in unprotected intercourse prior to the test, takes the test and then engages only in protected sex. The explanation given to this behavioural pattern is that testing facilitates behaviour change, that it 'works' as a means of HIV prevention. Secondly, the respondent engages in unprotected intercourse both before and after testing. The explanation given to this behavioural pattern is that the test has no impact, it does not 'work' as HIV prevention. However, there are two other behavioural patterns. Here respondents had not engaged in unprotected intercourse for some time (usually years) before testing. They reported behavioural change as occurring *prior* to the test. Following the test, they might continue to use condoms, either to protect themselves or others, or they might stop using them – usually because they were having sex with someone they knew or thought to be of the same HIV status (see below). It is the first two patterns, where testing follows at least one incident of unprotected intercourse, however, that will be the focus of the rest of the chapter.

Reasons for Only Protected Intercourse Following Testing

Some respondents had unprotected sex prior to the test but not in the time between testing and interview. When such apparent 'behaviour change' has been observed in research, commentators often assume it is due to testing. Our analysis indicates, however, that the impact of the test has been overestimated. For those who tested positive, consistent condom use was often due to fears of infecting others. In some cases these fears could lead to sexual problems or to avoiding sex altogether:

> When I knew for certain I was positive – and particularly having a
> sexual partner who was negative – I initially became a bit neurotic
> about keeping him protected . . . I was really, I suppose, quite scared
> and I think that affected my sexual performance to a degree by
> suddenly being very aware of my status and, you know, it almost

became too clinical at one stage. It was . . . to the point where I almost thought that I should stop seeing him cause I was so afraid of transmitting the virus to him. (Gay man, HIV+)

One 'safe' behavioural pattern after testing is thus no sex at all. Celibacy was only a deliberate risk reduction strategy for some positive respondents, however. In addition to fears of transmission to partners, celibacy could also be due to decreased sexual confidence, a loss of sexual pleasure, fears of rejection or negative reactions if they disclosed their HIV status to sexual partners, or the fact that diagnosis is such a significant and traumatizing event that sex – or any relationship at all – is the last thing wanted. Celibacy for some, however, was only a temporary response while coming to terms with diagnosis (Keogh, Beardsell and Sigma Research, 1997 obtained similar findings for gay men). HIV negative respondents, on the other hand, were rarely celibate as a risk reduction strategy. Instead, they tended not to have sex because of lack of opportunity or because of relationship problems at that time.

The stress of testing and a feeling that they could not put themselves through the experience again was often reported by HIV negative respondents as a reason for not having unprotected intercourse:

I've used safe sex [since the test] always. It was because I had a negative result and I just couldn't put myself through thinking again that I was positive. I just couldn't risk it, especially after escaping from drug using, it would be too much. (Heterosexual woman, HIV−)

However, some repeat testers reported that these feelings could dissipate with time:

I tend to be really good after the test. I'd even turn down money, a punter, I've even turned down a customer if he doesn't want to use a condom . . . and after a while, yeah, everything becomes more mellow you know, AIDS doesn't exist quite so strongly. (Heterosexual woman, HIV−)

Not wanting to infect others once diagnosed with HIV, and not wanting to put oneself at risk of infection again if HIV negative, are the common explanations given to consistent condom use by quantitative researchers. But two other explanations for so-called safe behaviour also emerged from our analysis, and this suggests that the impact of testing on behaviour might be overestimated. These explanations also illustrate the importance of considering the *meanings* that people attach to behaviours, not just the behaviours themselves.

Firstly, the behaviour that prompted testing may have been a one-off lapse from consistent condom use for some HIV negative respondents. They do not perceive themselves as having changed their behaviour from unsafe to safe at all – they see it as going back to how things were normally. Secondly, for some respondents, both positive and negative, behaviour change was not necessarily because of or wholly because of the test. They acknowledged that other factors were as important or more important:

> It's not just a question of whether you're negative or positive, life isn't that simple. When you've been for a test, that might seem the most monumental thing to do, but once you've passed through that there's a whole host of things to consider. And you still go out there and you're still an ordinary gay man out there on the scene or on the street or whatever, and you're still subject to the same unknown quantities of pressure, matched with your desires for sexual fulfil-ment and to be attractive and to attract. (Gay man, HIV−)

For some respondents, behaviour change was seen as part of a developmental process, something that would have happened anyway. Explanations included changes in drug use or involvement with the drug scene, in relationship status, in attitudes to sex, in responsibilities (such as parenthood), in social life (which might perhaps mean reduced opportunities for sex), or simply by getting older. Asked 'Have you changed your sexual behaviour in any way since the test?' one respondent said:

> Oh yeah ... well, just always using condoms, that's the only way really but ... it wasn't just that. I keep thinking that it's because I've grown up. I haven't had a relationship since. I've had short things, three months at the most, but I've reduced my sexual partners as well compared to before ... I'm sure [the test] did have some influence or whether you just change in your life. It's a whole sort of thing, you know, a combination of things. ... Just ... growing up as in, you know, discovering what you really need and how I don't necessarily possibly enjoy [sex] so much as I used to and it's not worth it as much – it's just what you get out of it, you know. When I was younger it was more important, now it's not so much of a big issue, if you like. I don't think it's because of the test but then again I also think that it has played a part in it as well. (Heterosexual woman, HIV+)

Reasons for Unprotected Intercourse Following Testing

Some people continue to have unprotected sex after testing. Why does testing appear to have no impact on their behaviour? Some apparently 'unsafe' re-spondents only had unprotected sex with someone they knew to be of the same HIV status. Such 'negotiated safety' (Kippax *et al.*, 1992) was fairly common among HIV negative respondents:

Monogamy is the big condom for both of us. (Gay man, HIV−)

A test was often taken so that couples could dispense with condoms. Most heterosexuals saw negotiated safety as relatively unproblematic and some felt that it was safer than using condoms, which they thought unreliable. It was only a few gay men who raised any concerns about the safety of negotiated safety:

That's still a kind of evolving thing, the commitment issue. If we can rely on that ... know that the two of us are safe enough to have unsafe sex ... as long as we're faithful to each other, then that's a different situation altogether. It's an enormously difficult problem. It goes on endlessly because so much of it is based on what isn't seen and what isn't known or can't be scrutinized or understood fully. So, I mean, I see myself as being safe and being in a safe situation but at the same time I don't think it is ... because I can't have all the information 'cause there's this limit to how much you can know of somebody else's choice and where they've been and where they want to be. (Gay man, HIV−)

Some respondents with HIV had unprotected sex with other HIV positive people. Positive partners were often preferred because this avoided fears of transmitting infection to others or adverse reactions to disclosure. However, for some, decisions about whether to have unprotected sex with someone could be based on assumptions or informed guesses about their serostatus, not necessarily the certainty that they are also HIV positive:

Some people talk about negotiating safer sex. There has only been a couple of occasions when we've sat down and said, 'Look I'm positive, you're positive, d'you wanna use a condom?' 'No'. 'Is there any point?' 'No'. 'Let's go ahead and have unsafe sex'.' Sometimes, if I've told the person that I'm about to have unsafe sex with that I'm positive and if we continue and have sex and we don't use a condom and if I feel that they themselves know what they're doing, then we go ahead – not having negotiated – yes, we go ahead and have unsafe sex, we do it anyway. . . . Sometimes when I'm telling them that I'm positive, they'll say, 'I'm positive as well.' It may be somebody that I know to be positive or actually, the majority of times that it happens is somebody I've told I'm positive, they haven't told me what their status is but they have continued with unsafe sex . . . and they start to fuck me without a condom and I've just continued with it basically. So, to me, it's been their decision and, I mean, if it was somebody that I sort of thought to myself they know nothing about the gay scene, they know nothing about what is safe, what isn't, then I wouldn't do it. It's people that I know would know, if that makes sense. (Gay man, HIV+)

This was linked to the theme that it is the responsibility of both partners to ensure the safety of sexual encounters, and the onus should not be exclusively on the HIV positive partner, although this was a minority view.

Some respondents had unprotected sex because they disliked condoms or had difficulties using them, and some women experienced difficulties always negotiating safer sex or were not necessarily in control of condom use. However, HIV positive respondents were much more likely to work successfully at overcoming these problems. The other themes associated with no condom or inconsistent condom use after testing emerged only from the discourses of HIV negative respondents.

Spontaneity and passion were fairly common explanations for unsafe sex. Some respondents, mainly heterosexual, assessed risk in terms of 'it's not what you do it's who you do it with'. Unprotected sex is only perceived as risky if their partner is perceived as 'risky', e.g. someone who has injected drugs or just used them, someone from a high risk country, a bisexual or 'promiscuous' person. Respondents might see the test as changing their behaviour in terms of being more 'choosy' about their partners, so they would only use condoms with more 'risky' ones; by 'getting to know' their partners better before they have unprotected sex with them; or by reducing partner numbers:

> Not 100 per cent but I am more cautious I would say . . . I'm more likely to insist on a guy using a condom but it depends who it is sometimes. . . . If I know someone quite intimately, like it might be an old boyfriend that I've known for a few years, I might be more relaxed with them but if it's somebody I don't know then I will. (Heterosexual woman, HIV−)

R I think [I'd have another test] maybe if I found out that one of my partners since then that I'd had unprotected sex with had sex with someone (a) obviously who was HIV positive, or (b) who was in a high risk category or what I perceive to be a high risk category.

I Which is?

R Drug users, homosexuals, prostitutes, promiscuous − promiscuity . . . and also probably how many partners I've had unprotected sex with − of which I've had two since them.

I How many partners would count as enough?

R I don't know. It would be something that would creep up on me, you know. I did consider it again quite recently, actually. I thought about it [but] it hasn't become enough of a wave in my head yet. (Heterosexual man, HIV−)

Consistent condom use could also be a problem for female sex workers who might be in a particularly vulnerable position and might get paid more for unprotected sex:

> They won't say yes to a condom. The number of times I've got beaten up badly. . . . This guy, I turned round and before I turn around he's got the Durex off his dick. (Heterosexual woman, HIV−)

They might also associate condom use with work not pleasure:

> The thing that puts me off is that I equate it with work, so I really have a problem with it. I think, 'No, I really like it, this is for my pleasure.'. . . I'd even get them out, open the packet and not use it. Or the slightest bit of 'ooh' from them I'd say, 'Oh go on, take it off, don't worry.' And that was ridiculous but that's how it is. (Heterosexual woman, HIV−)

Finally, some respondents could find no other explanation for their behaviour than that it was somehow out of their control. They described their behaviour as 'irresponsible' but saw unsafe sex as inevitable and thus repeat testing as inevitable:

> I'm ashamed to admit it to you, I'm so ashamed to say I haven't really changed my sexual behaviour . . . I'm exposing myself to this thing because I'm not using, like, barrier contraception. I mean, I'm sorry to say it but I haven't changed my behaviour. . . . Maybe it's the sort of person I am that brings me to the clinic in the first place and possibly the sort of person I am means that there's every chance I'm going to be going for a third test. (Heterosexual woman, HIV−)

Discussion

There has often been an assumption made by researchers, policy makers and other commentators that the relationship between behaviour prior to testing, the decision to have a test and behaviour after testing is linear: an awareness that engaging in unprotected sex carries the risk of HIV transmission leads to having an HIV test to check if infection has occurred, which in turns leads to behaviour change to protect themselves or their sexual partners, depending on the result. The present chapter, however, has illustrated that these relationships are more complex than has been assumed. Testing is not an immediate response to risk, and the levels of risk perceived as risky enough to warrant an HIV test vary across individuals. Thus the baseline against which behaviour can change is not uniform. Changes in behaviour after having a test are not necessarily solely (or even partly) due to testing, and there are a whole range of other factors which can impact more strongly on sexual behaviour. For instance, diagnosis with HIV can have an enormous impact on sexuality. While this has been observed in research before (e.g. McKegany, 1990; Pergami *et al.*, 1993; Green, 1994; Jones, Klimes and Catalan, 1994; Remien, Carballo-Diéguez and Wagner, 1995; Keogh, Beardsell and Sigma Research, 1997), such findings have not been considered when explaining the behavioural impact of HIV testing. Similarly, research investigating unprotected intercourse in general HIV negative (mainly untested) samples have found similar reasons or rationales for not using condoms. These include a dislike of condoms (e.g. Holland *et al.*, 1990; Maticka-Tyndale, 1992; Davies *et al.*, 1993; Molenaar, Hospers and Kok, 1993; White *et al.*, 1993; Lowy and Ross, 1994; Maxwell and Boyle, 1994; Quirk and Rhodes, 1995); a belief that condoms are unreliable (e.g. Maticka-Tyndale, 1992; Weiss, Weston and Quirindale, 1993; Choi, Rickman and Catania, 1994); gendered power relations and difficulties negotiating condom use (e.g. Holland *et al.*, 1990, 1991, 1992; White *et al.*, 1993; Kippax, Crawford and Walby, 1994; Maxwell and Boyle, 1994); love and passion (e.g. Kippax *et al.*, 1990; Prieur, 1990; Davies *et al.*, 1993; de Wit *et al.*, 1994; Lowy and Ross, 1994; Quirk and Rhodes, 1995); selecting 'safe' partners (e.g. Maticka-Tyndale, 1992; Kippax, Crawford and Walby, 1994; Lowy and Ross, 1994); and a reliance on trust and monogamy or discarding condoms once a relationship is established (e.g. Maticka-Tyndale, 1992; Wight, 1992; Davies *et al.*, 1993; de Wit *et al.*, 1994; Kippax, Crawford and Walby, 1994; Maxwell and Boyle, 1994). The fact that similar themes emerge in the present study suggests that the impact of the test has been overestimated and that the test is not 'powerful' enough to change behaviour in the face of these other factors, sometimes even for those who test HIV positive.

The rationales for behaviour after testing indicate the importance of studying the meanings that individuals attach to their behaviour, not just the behaviours themselves. Epidemiological categories of risk are not identical to risk perceptions, but it is the perceptions that determine behaviour (Lowy and Ross, 1994). For example, the use of 'negotiated safety' or partner selection as prevention strategies may not be foolproof but respondents perceived them as such, and testing does not necessarily have any impact on such perceptions. Further research might concentrate on how pre- and post-test counselling sessions might be used to better effect here, particularly since respondents did not believe these sessions had any impact on behaviour.

Knowledge of HIV status can inform behaviour but may be only one of a range of factors taken into account. HIV testing is thus not a 'magic bullet' which automatically leads to behaviour change. While there may be a range of benefits to the individual of testing, this research suggests that to promote testing on the basis of public health benefits is unwarranted. Many HIV positive respondents in this study did not think that their behaviour had placed them at significant risk. More public health benefit might be gained from health promotion aimed at improving the accuracy of individuals' risk assessments. The HIV test is a diagnostic tool not an intervention, and should only be 'promoted' as part of an individuals risk reduction strategy, not as an end in itself.

References

ALLEN, S., SERUFILIRA, A., GRUBER, V., KEGELES, S., VAN DE PERRE, P., CARAEL, M. and COATES, T.J. (1993) 'Pregnancy and contraceptive use among urban Rwandan women after HIV testing and counselling', *American Journal of Public Health*, **83**, pp. 705–10.

BEARDSELL, S. (1994) 'Should wider HIV testing be encouraged on the grounds of HIV prevention?', *AIDS Care*, **6**, 1, pp. 5–19.

BEARDSELL, S. and COYLE, A. (1996) 'A review of research on the nature and quality of HIV testing services: a proposal for process-based studies', *Social Science and Medicine*, **42**, 5, pp. 733–43.

BEARDSELL, S., HICKSON, F.C.I. and WEATHERBURN, P. (1995) *HIV Testing Services in North Thames (East)*. London: North Thames Regional Health Authority and Sigma Research.

BEEVOR, A.S. and CATALAN, J. (1993) 'Women's experiences of HIV testing: the views of HIV positive and HIV negative women', *AIDS Care*, **5**, 2, pp. 177–86.

CHOI, K.H., RICKMAN, R. and CATANIA, J.A. (1994) 'What heterosexual adults believe about condoms', *New England Journal of Medicine*, **331**, 6, pp. 406–7.

DAVIES, P.M., HICKSON, F.C.I., WEATHERBURN, P. and HUNT, A.J. (1993) *Sex, Gay Men and AIDS*. London: Falmer Press.

DELGADO-RODRIGUEZ, M., DE LA FUENTE, L., BRAVO, M.J., LARDELLI, P. and BARRIO, G. (1994) 'IV drug users: changes in risk behaviour according to HIV status in a national survey in Spain', *Journal of Epidemiology and Community Health*, **24**, pp. 463–69.

DESENCLOS, J.G., PAPAEVANGELOU, G. and ANCELLE-PARK, R. (1993) 'Knowledge of HIV serostatus and preventative behaviour among European injecting drug users', *AIDS*, **7**, pp. 1371–77.

DOLL, L.S. and KENNEDY, M.B. (1994) 'HIV counselling and testing: What is it and how well does it work?', in Schochtetman, G. and George, J.R. (eds) *AIDS Testing: A Comprehensive Guide to Technical, Medical, Social, Legal and Management Issues*. New York: Springer-Vale.

GLASER, B. and STRAUSS, A. (1967) *The Discovery of Grounded Theory*. Chicago, IL: Aldine.

GREEN, G. (1994) 'Positive sex: sexual relationships following an HIV diagnosis', in Aggleton, P., Davies, P. and Hart, G. (eds) *AIDS: Foundations for the Future*. London: Taylor & Francis.

HIGGINS, D.L., GALAVOTTI, C., O'REILLEY, K.R. *et al.* (1991) 'Evidence of the effects of HIV and antibody counselling and testing on risk behaviors', *Journal of the American Medical Association*, **226**, pp. 2419–29.

HOLLAND, J., RAMAZANOGLU, C., SCOTT, S., SHARPE, S. and THOMPSON, R. (1990) 'Sex, gender and power: young women's sexuality in the shadow of AIDS', *Sociology of Health and Illness*, **12**, pp. 336–50.

HOLLAND, J., RAMAZANOGLU, C., SCOTT, S., SHARPE, S. and THOMPSON, R. (1991) 'Between embarrassment and trust: young women and the diversity of condom use', in Aggleton, P., Davies, P. and Hart, G. (eds) *AIDS: Responses, Interventions and Care.* London: Taylor & Francis.

HOLLAND, J., RAMAZANOGLU, C., SCOTT, S., SHARPE, S. and THOMPSON, R. (1992) 'Risk, power and the possibility of pleasure: young women and safer sex', *AIDS Care*, **4**, pp. 273–83.

ICKOVICS, J.R., MORRILL, A.C., BEREN, S.E., WALSH, U. and RODIN, J. (1994) 'Limited effects of HIV counselling and testing for women: a prospective study of behavioral and psychological consequences', *Journal of the American Medical Association*, **272**, 6, pp. 443–48.

DES JARLAIS, C.C., FRIEDMAN, S.R., FRIEDMAN, P., WENSTON, J., SOTHERAN, J.L., CHOOPANYA, K., VANICHSENI, S., RAKTHAM, S., GOLDBERG, D., FRISCHER, M., GREEN, S., LIMA, E.L., BASTOS, F.I. and TELLES, P.R. (1995) 'HIV/AIDS-related behavior change among injecting drug users in different national settings', *AIDS*, **9**, pp. 611–17.

JONES, M., KLIMES, I. and CATALAN, J.J. (1994) 'Psychosexual problems in people with HIV infection: controlled study of gay men and men with haemophilia', *AIDS Care*, **6**, 5, pp. 587–93.

KELLY, J.A. MURPHY, D.A. and BAHR, G.R. (1993) 'Factors associated with the severity of depression in high risk sexual behaviour amongst persons diagnosed with human immunodeficiency virus (HIV)', *Health Psychology*, **12**, 3, pp. 215–19.

KEOGH, P., BEARDSELL, S. and SIGMA RESEARCH (1997) 'Sexual negotiation strategies of HIV-positive gay men: a qualitative investigation', in Aggleton, P., Davies, P. and Hart, G. (eds) *AIDS: Activism and Alliances.* London: Taylor and Francis.

KIPPAX, S., CRAWFORD, J. and WALBY, C. (1994) 'Heterosexuality, masculinity and HIV', *AIDS*, **8**, suppl. 1, pp. 315–23.

KIPPAX, S., CRAWFORD, J., WALBY, C. and BENTON, P. (1990) 'Women negotiating heterosex: implications for AIDS prevention', *Womens Studies International Forum*, **13**, pp. 533–42.

KIPPAX, S., DOWSETT, G.W., DAVIES, M., RODDEN, P. and CRAWFORD, J. (1992) 'Sustaining safer sex or relapse: gay men's responses to HIV'. Paper presented at the VIIIth International Conference on AIDS, Amsterdam (TuD 0545).

Lowy, E. and Ross, M.W. (1994) '"It'll never happen to me': gay men's beliefs, perceptions and folk constructions of sexual risk', *AIDS Education and Prevention*, **6**, 6, pp. 467–82.

McKeganey, N. (1990) 'Being positive: drug injectors' experiences of being HIV positive', *British Journal of Addiction*, **85**, 1113–24.

Maticka-Tyndale, E. (1992) 'Social construction of HIV transmission and prevention among heterosexual young adults', *Social Problems*, **39**, 3, pp. 238–52.

Maxwell, C. and Boyle, M. (1994) 'Risky heterosexual practices amongst women over 30: gender, power and long-term relationships', *AIDS Care*, **7**, 3, pp. 277–93.

Molenaar, S., Hospers, H. and Kok, G. (1993) 'Why do some gay men engage in risk-taking sex and how should the field of health education react to this?'. Paper presented at the 7th Conference on Social Aspects of AIDS, London.

Pergami, A., Gala, C., Burgess, A., Durbano, F., Zanello, D., Riccio, M., Invernizzi, G. and Catalan, J. (1993) 'The psychosocial impact of HIV infection in women', *Journal of Psychosomatic Research*, **37**, 7, pp. 687–96.

Pickering, H., Quigley, M., Pépin, J., Todd, J. and Wilkins, A. (1993) 'The effects of post-test counselling on condom use among prostitutes in the Gambia', *AIDS*, **7**, pp. 271–73.

Prieur, A. (1990) 'Norwegian gay men: reasons for continued practice of unsafe sex', *AIDS Education and Prevention*, **2**, pp. 109–15.

Quirk, A. and Rhodes, T. (1995) 'Condom use by drug users: whether, why not and how?', *Executive Summary 41*. London: CRDHB.

Remien, R.H., Carballo-Diéguez, A. and Wagner, G. (1995) 'Intimacy and sexual risk behaviour in serodiscordant male couples', *AIDS Care*, **7**, 4, pp. 429–38.

Roffman, R.A., Kalichman, S.C., Kelly, J.A., Winett, R.A., Solomon, L.J., Sikkema. K.J., Norman, A.D., Desiderato, L.L., Perry, M.J., Lemke, A.L., Steiner, S. and Stevenson, L.Y. (1995) 'HIV antibody testing of gay men in smaller US cities', *AIDS Care*, **7**, 4, pp. 405–13.

Strauss, A. and Corbin, J. (1990) *Basics of Qualitative Research: Grounded Theory Procedures and Techniques*. Newbury Park, CA: Sage.

Weiss, S.H., Weston, C.B. and Quirindale, J. (1993) 'Safe sex? Misconceptions, gender differences and barriers among injection drug users: a focus group approach', *AIDS Education and Prevention*, **5**, 4, pp. 279–93.

Wenger, N.S., Kusseling, F.S., Beck, K. and Shapiro, M.F. (1994) 'When patients first suspect and find out they are infected with the human immunodeficiency virus: implications for prevention', *AIDS Care*, **6**, 4, pp. 399–405.

White, D., Phillips, K., Mulleady, G. and Cupitt, C. (1993) 'Sexual issues and condom use among injecting drug users'. *AIDS Care*, **5**, 4, pp. 427–37.

WIGHT, D. (1992) 'Impediments to safer heterosexual sex: a review of research with young people', *AIDS Care*, **4**, pp. 11–23.

DE WIT, J.B.F., TUENIS, N., VAN GRIENSVEN, G.J.P. and SANDFORT, T. (1994) 'Behavioral risk-reduction strategies to prevent HIV infection among homosexual men: a grounded theory approach', *AIDS Education and Prevention*, **6**, 6, pp. 493–505.

WOLITSKI, R., MACGOWAN, R., HIGGINS, D. and JORGENSEN, C. (1997) *AIDS Education and Prevention*, **9**, suppl. B, pp. 52–67.

ZAPKA, J.G., STODDARD, A., ZORN, M.M., McCUSKER, J. and MAYER, K.H. (1991) 'HIV antibody test result knowledge, risk perceptions and behaviour among homosexually active men', *Patient Education and Counselling*, **18**, pp. 9–17.

Chapter 13

Treatment Education: A Multidisciplinary Challenge

Will Anderson and Peter Weatherburn

The advent of anti-HIV combination therapy has changed the lives of many people living with HIV and offers hope to many more. Yet given the complexity of treatment options, the difficulties of managing the therapies and the lack of any data on the long-term consequences of therapy, any individual's decision to start therapy remains difficult. Our understanding of how individuals make such choices remains very limited.

One of the key concerns for people with HIV in the new clinical environment – where treatment options are compelling but complex – is their own knowledge about HIV treatment and therapy and the information available to them. This chapter presents data about the treatment information and education needs of people living with HIV in the United Kingdom. The research, carried out by the National AIDS Manual (NAM) with Sigma Research, provides an insight into the experience of people with HIV in obtaining and using treatments information. The results of this research suggest that a differentiated and multidisciplinary approach is needed to meet the challenges of HIV treatment education – a task which will always be complex and require different inputs at different times.

The Clinical and the Social

When negotiating their treatment and therapy choices, people with HIV must deal with a variety of social tasks. These include getting access to appropriate services and assessing the quality of those services; building relationships with doctors and other health professionals; obtaining and assessing information about available treatments; gaining the understanding and confidence to make fully informed decisions; managing the impact of treatment regimens on daily life and personal relationships; and dealing with the longer-term impact of starting treatment – on individual identity, life plans and work prospects.

The relatively slow progress of clinical research during much of the HIV epidemic has discouraged social researchers from engaging with these social tasks, especially when HIV prevention seemed to offer so many fruitful opportunities for inquiry. The professional divisions between clinical practice and social science have also acted as a disincentive to social inquiry into treatment issues.

Now that medicine has much more to offer people with HIV, the case for research which investigates the social demands of clinical success is much more persuasive. Furthermore, the renewed professional interest in treatment access, education and compliance presents questions about who should be taking responsibility for these social tasks as well as what form they should take.

Although these issues have been given a new urgency by the recent clinical results, questions about access, education, informed consent, compliance and the social determinants of personal well-being have a longer history, particularly in the attempts by people with HIV to shape a clinical culture in which they are involved as equal partners, not as subordinate patients. The history of HIV treatment activism (in all its forms) provides a strong foundation on which to build contemporary personal and professional responses to the opportunities of the new therapies.

Understanding the Tasks of HIV Treatment Education

The lack of research into the social aspects of HIV treatment means that professionals must pursue their work without a rigorous understanding of the knowledge, experience, expectations and needs of people with HIV in accessing and using treatments. As combination therapy becomes an integral part of the lives of people with HIV in the UK, the need for such research is likely to become more pressing.

Existing research in HIV treatment education is almost exclusively concerned with the evaluation of particular projects. These include published resources (Guimento *et al.*, 1994; McLanahan *et al.*, 1994; Korsia and Majchrowicz, 1994; Kuromiya and Bauer, 1996; Baker and Copeland, 1996), helplines (Mark, 1994; Katz *et al.*, 1996; Nalbandian *et al.*, 1996), community initiatives and peer education (McClure *et al.*, 1996; Pleasant *et al.*, 1996; Brown, 1996). Most of these studies originate in North America, although some projects (e.g. Thomas, 1994) have inspired similar initiatives in the UK.

What is clearly lacking from this literature is research which attempts to investigate the experience of people with HIV independent of any particular intervention. In 1996 NAM undertook such an investigation: a needs assessment of the treatment information needs of people living with HIV. The aim of the study was to obtain a better understanding of the treatment information needs of people living with HIV in the UK and to assess the role of existing treatment information resources in meeting those needs. The term 'treatment information resources' encompassed both published and human resources.

This research was undertaken immediately prior to the Vancouver AIDS Conference in July 1996, which triggered international interest in combination anti-HIV therapies. It therefore provides a baseline account of how people with HIV engage with treatment issues in general and with treatment information and education in particular.

Methods and Sample

The study employed a four-sided self-complete questionnaire, designed to obtain a broad range of quantitative information from a large number of people living with HIV. A draft was piloted and other treatment information providers were consulted. Inevitably, there were competing demands of content and brevity.

The questionnaire was distributed in March 1996 through two mechanisms: batches were sent to genito-urinary medicine (GUM) clinics, drop-in centres and other AIDS service organizations; and they were included in mailings of *AIDS Treatment Update, Body Positive Newsletter, Continuum* magazine and *Mainliners Newsletter.*

There were 751 respondents, of whom 90% were men. The sample was also overwhelmingly White; Black and Asian ethnic groups accounted for only just over 5% of the sample. Three-quarters (76%) of the respondents identified as gay men and one-fifth as heterosexual (19%). Almost half (49%) lived in Greater London with the remainder drawn from three-quarters of all the 124 postcode regions in the UK. The mean age was 38, with a range from 16 to 66. Three-quarters (75%) had experienced some HIV-related symptoms and just under one-third (31%) had received an AIDS diagnosis.

There were two substantial differences between the sample and national data on people diagnosed with HIV: the underrepresentation of Black Africans and a relatively high proportion of symptomatic respondents. Only 2.1% of the sample identified as Black African (with another 1.2% identifying themselves as Black 'other' and 0.3% Black Caribbean) compared to 13.9% of people diagnosed with HIV nationally.[1] This underrepresentation undoubtedly reflects less access to the newsletters and resources that formed the basis of the recruitment strategy. It may also be partly due to lower levels of literacy in English. There is clearly a need for targeted research into experiences of accessing treatment within this population group, which represents almost one in seven of those living with HIV in the UK.

The proportion of symptomatic respondents was 44% compared to 35% nationally.[2] Given that the questionnaire addressed treatment issues, it is not surprising that a greater proportion of symptomatic people with HIV returned it than those diagnosed but asymptomatic.

Four issues arising from the data are discussed in the remainder of this chapter: reasons for starting or not starting anti-HIV therapy; sources of HIV treatment information; knowledge of HIV medicine; and the role of doctors.

Reasons for Starting Anti-HIV Therapy

The use of anti-HIV drugs remains somewhat controversial in the UK. Questions about the efficacy, side effects and sustainability of anti-HIV drugs have always dominated public discussion of their value. This inevitably makes life difficult for those facing the choice of whether or not to take these drugs. Unfortunately, the quality of debates about anti-HIV drugs has not always helped. The *a priori* opposition to any form of anti-HIV treatment taken by some commentators did nothing to increase the confidence of those making treatment decisions.

However, recent clinical advances have swept away most of the old doubts about therapies and the question now faced by most people with HIV is when, not if, they should start taking therapy. Although the survey was undertaken before any widespread publicity about the efficacy of combination therapy, treatment news about anti-HIV therapy had been increasingly optimistic for over a year.

Respondents were asked whether or not they had ever taken anti-HIV therapy and to identify the reasons for their choice. Those who had taken such treatments may have been reflecting on decisions taken years earlier. Three-fifths (61%) had taken some form of anti-HIV drug. Predictably, more symptomatic respondents (68%) had taken anti-HIV drugs than asymptomatic respondents (39%). Similarly, more of those with an AIDS diagnosis (85%) had taken anti-HIV drugs than those without an AIDS diagnosis (50%). There were no associations between respondents' experience of taking anti-HIV drugs and their sex, ethnicity, sexuality or place of residence.

The respondents who had not taken any anti-HIV drugs were asked to tick any of six reasons why they had not done so. They could tick as many as applied to them. The 298 respondents who had not taken anti-HIV drugs gave 501 reasons. Table 13.1 describes the percentage of respondents who identified each reason for not having taken anti-HIV drugs and provides an analysis across the stages of illness.

Not surprisingly, as people experience symptoms or receive an AIDS diagnosis, the proportion who continue not to take anti-HIV drugs tend to do so for increasingly critical reasons. In particular, the assessment that the benefits are not worth the side effects was made by almost two-thirds (63%) of the respondents with AIDS who had decided not to start therapy, whereas this reason was given by only one-quarter of the asymptomatic respondents. Respondents who had taken anti-HIV drugs were asked to tick any of five possible reasons why they had first chosen to start taking them. Again, they could tick all that applied. The 458 respondents who had taken anti-HIV drugs gave a total of 805 reasons. Table 13.2 lists the percentage of respondents who identified each reason for having first taken anti-HIV drugs. The role of doctors in shaping decisions to start anti-HIV treatment is clear. However, although two-thirds of those who had taken anti-HIV drugs identified doctors' advice as a reason for doing so, this leaves one-third who did not identify their

Table 13.1   Reasons for choosing not to take anti-HIV drugs

Reason	Percentage of respondents who had not taken anti-HIV drugs			
	All	Asymptomatic	Symptomatic	AIDS
I have been well and haven't needed to	69	82	60	43
I decided that the benefits are not worth the risk of side effects	36	25	44	63
I have heard/read bad reports about them	32	25	36	46
I don't think they work	20	17	24	37
My doctor recommended not to	9	9	9	6
The drugs have not been available when I wanted them	2	2	2	3

doctor's advice as an influence on their decision. From the perspective of the traditional medical model, this is a more surprising result.

Considered together, the results from these two questions have a number of interesting features. First, the assessment of the costs and benefits of taking anti-HIV drugs played an equally important role for those who chose to take anti-HIV drugs as it did for those who chose not to. However, reading or hearing bad reports about treatments influenced almost one-third of those who did not take anti-HIV drugs, whereas good reports were much less influential for those who did take them (16%). This may be because bad news is more keenly heard by those who it may impact on, or that bad news is more widely reported. Either way, the task of giving people with HIV a full and honest picture of the costs and benefits of treatments is not a simple one; in particular, the reporting of 'bad' news about drugs should always be always qualified as rigorously as the reporting of 'good' news.

Secondly, similar perceptions of health status lead to completely different treatment decisions. Seven out of ten of those who had not taken anti-HIV drugs felt that their good health did not warrant starting therapy, whereas three out of ten of those who had taken anti-HIV drugs did so because they wanted to maintain their good health.

The pressure to intervene early with anti-HIV drugs (i.e. before the onset of illness) has grown considerably since the survey was undertaken. But even if the clinical rationale for doing this is stronger, the psychological (as well as practical) difficulties of starting complex treatment regimens when healthy

Table 13.2   Reasons for choosing to take anti-HIV drugs

Reason	Percentage of respondents who had taken anti-HIV drugs
My doctor recommended it/told me to	68
I decided that the benefits were worth the risk of side effects	37
I had become ill	29
I was well and wanted to stay that way	26
I had heard/read good reports about it	16

should not be underestimated. If starting treatment has been seen by some as the defining moment of illness, changes in the clinical use of therapies may need to be accompanied by more profound changes in how therapy is perceived in relation to health and illness. Recent qualitative work on the impact of combination therapies (Anderson and Weatherburn, 1996) has described the emergence of a range of new 'stories' about therapy which are displacing the discouraging stories of the past – but individual interpretation of these stories remains complex.

Sources of HIV Treatment Information

People living with HIV have had to deal with a unique range of problems in obtaining reliable information about treatments, including the misinformation put out by a sensationalist media and the radical differences of opinion among community organizations. Consequently, the range and importance of information sources is likely to be different from the experience of those with other illnesses.

A key aim of the survey was to map the resources which people living with HIV use. Twenty-one information sources were listed in the questionnaire in random order. Figure 13.1 shows, for each information source, the percentage who said the source was very important, quite important and not at all important to them in developing their knowledge of HIV treatments and medicine. The sources are in descending order of frequency of selection of the 'very important' category.

These results are encouraging in that they suggest people are getting treatment information from a wide and diverse range of places. The diversity is important. Note the top three very important sources: HIV newsletters, doctors and positive people. Each of them has a very different claim to authority. Newsletters enjoy the authority of the printed word; doctors have the authority of professional training; and people living with HIV have the authority of experience. The fact that all three are considered to be important sources

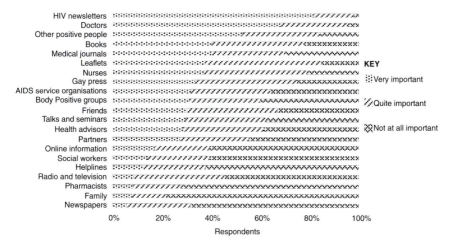

Figure 13.1 HIV: sources of treatment information and their importance.

of HIV treatment information suggests that many people with HIV have been able to develop their own critical perspective on treatment information by viewing it from very different perspectives.

The majority of information resources were identified as being very important by 30–40% of respondents. Published information is again prominent, with books, medical journals, leaflets and the gay press all widely used. Among the human resources, professionals, both in statutory and voluntary settings, are given similar ratings to the informal educators of partners and friends.

Among the group of resources which are used least, the national media is prominent: radio, television and particularly the newspapers were rarely considered to be very important. However, many more Black respondents (21%) than White respondents (5%) said that newspapers were very important. Perhaps the most surprising category included at this level is pharmacists, a profession with a clear brief for treatment education. Pharmacists are likely to play an increasingly important role in treatment education, given the importance of compliance to the new combination regimens.

Three qualifications need to be made to the generally optimistic picture presented by these results. First, some of the scores are actually not very high, given the specialist nature of the services concerned. Only one in three said that AIDS service organizations had been very important to them, and only one in eight felt that helplines had been very important. Second, although these results indicate the potential for a wide range of services to be involved in treatment education, they do not actually tell us anything about how many are actively pursuing this work. For example, it would take only one communicative doctor in an otherwise terrible HIV outpatient clinic to produce (locally) a good result. Thirdly, these results say nothing about the quality of the information obtained. This is a crucial issue, especially in the current environment where relatively complex questions of compliance and cross-resistance are so important to the success of treatment regimens. Also, the data does not tell us anything about the relative importance of different sources of information to particular individuals. Notwithstanding these qualifications, the results do suggest that a diversity of people in a diversity of contexts are contributing to treatment education for people with HIV.

Addressing the social aspects of treatment will always require a multidisciplinary approach. The data tells us nothing about the extent of collaboration or common strategy between different agencies or different professionals. But they indicate the potential for such strategy. The danger remains that the lack of professional ownership of responsibility for treatment education will lead to a lack of strategic development. Doctors are first and foremost clinicians not educators and, although they clearly pay a crucial role in treatment education, there will continue to be a need for a more diverse response to the needs of people with HIV. Whether this is possible in the current competitive provider environment remains to be seen.

Knowledge of HIV Medicine

Any response to the treatment education needs of people with HIV should begin with a consideration of what those needs are. Hence the study sought to map out respondents' knowledge of HIV treatments and medicine, albeit in a very rudimentary way, in order to obtain an indication of the range of methods (and expertise) that treatment education needs to encompass.

The survey aimed to get a basic measure of respondents' knowledge about HIV and AIDS medicine by asking whether they knew, did not know, or were not sure about ten statements relating to HIV treatment. It was difficult to design because a 'true or false' test – with its inevitable risk of confusing people – would have been unethical. Hence the format relied on the frankness of respondents in stating their prior knowledge about each of the statements. The results are likely to suggest a higher level of knowledge than would have been recorded with a test in which 'answers' were not given.

The statements ranged from fairly basic to more technical or specialist. They were designed to be uncontroversial, but inevitably not everyone agreed that all were true. Although there was no category for disagreement, some respondents made it clear they did not agree with some statements. Figure 13.2 lists the statements and responses to them.

Not surprisingly, questions about the common practicalities of treatment were often known; for example, 'Septrin is widely used as PCP prophylaxis' was known by 86% of respondents. But the more technical questions were only known by a minority; for example, 'PCR tests look for virus rather than antibodies' was only known by 25%.

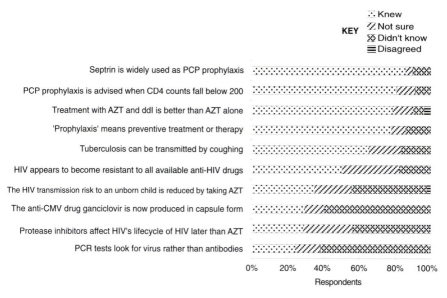

Figure 13.2   Knowledge of HIV medicine and therapy (ddI is dideoxyinosine).

However, quite substantial numbers of respondents did not know about some of the more basic questions of HIV treatment; for example, 22% did not know or were not sure that 'prophylaxis means preventive treatment'. In addition, it is arguable that even the more technical questions were not that advanced or specialist, yet 'the risk of transmission of HIV to an unborn child can be reduced by taking AZT' was known by only 35% (although by more women than men).

The key point here, once again, is diversity. About 5% of respondents knew only one out of ten and about 5% knew them all, with a very predictable distribution in between. This diversity needs to be reflected in the provision of treatment education; these results do not provide an argument for one kind of intervention over another.

There will always be people seeking technical, sophisticated information, just as there will always be people seeking very basic introductions to the subject. Similarly, although educators should always think very hard about how they can make their work accessible to as wide a range of people as possible, they should not assume that everything must be geared to those with the lowest levels of knowledge or understanding.

The Role of Doctors

Doctors have already featured prominently in this discussion of HIV treatment education. They play a central role in treatment decision making and are

Table 13.3   Attitudes to doctors

	Percentage of respondents agreeing with statement
My doctor is well informed about HIV and AIDS	88
My doctor listens to what I say	82
My doctor explains the choices I have about the treatments available	70
My doctor makes treatment decisions with me rather than for me	70

important sources of treatment information to many (though not all) people with HIV. However, these results do not necessarily reflect good relationships between doctors and people with HIV. The questionnaire attempted to address this issue by asking respondents to support a series of statements about their doctors. Table 13.3 lists the statements with the proportion of respondents who agreed with each.

Overall the confidence shown in doctors was high: a substantial majority agreed with each statement. However, given the importance of doctors in treatment choices, the experience of the minority of respondents is important: one in eight did not think that their doctor was well informed; more than one in six did not think that their doctor listened to what they said; almost one-third did not think their doctor explained the choices they had about treatments available; and almost one-third did not think their doctor made treatment decisions with them rather than for them.

Furthermore, there were strong associations between the satisfaction shown in doctors and whether respondents identified them as being a very important source of information. Basically, if a respondent revealed that they had a good relationship with their doctor, they were much more likely to identify doctors as being a very important source of information. For example, of the respondents who said their doctor was well informed about HIV and AIDS, 72% had identified doctors as a very important source of information. However, of the respondents who did not think their doctor was well informed about HIV and AIDS, only 39% identified their doctor as a very important source of information. This pattern is repeated for each of the questions about the quality of doctor relationships.

That doctors who explain treatment choices are perceived to be important sources of information is not very surprising. However, those who had good relationships with their doctors also had higher levels of knowledge about HIV treatments and medicine. Respondents who said their doctor was well informed about HIV and AIDS had a higher knowledge score (average 57%) than those who did not (49%). This pattern is repeated for all the questions about the quality of doctor relationships, except for the last.

Whether or not respondents' doctors listened to them did not (predictably) relate to their own knowledge level.

These results are encouraging, but they emphasize that the problems faced by those who do not have a good relationship with their doctor are all the more pressing. This is important for treatment educators in thinking about the aims and scope of their tasks. Supporting people in developing successful and fruitful relationships with their doctors should be a key task. However, both the importance and the limitations of what doctors can do in educating and informing their patients needs to be acknowledged.

Conclusions

The diversity of treatment information needs of people with HIV needs to be recognized, respected and addressed. For those engaged in HIV treatment education, the constant supply-side pressures – the endless stream of new information to be disseminated – can dull the senses to the plurality of the demand among people with HIV. This research provides an insight into this plurality. People with HIV will always need a very wide range of educational interventions from basic information to complex analysis. In turn, this range of interventions will require input from all the professionals and agencies with a concern for the clinical experience of people with HIV. Treatment education need not be the concern of a few experts.

As the clinical implications of combination therapy become clearer, research is needed into the diversity of personal and social issues faced by people with HIV before and after choosing to start therapy. Further evaluation of the increasing amount of treatment information and the growing number of educational initiatives should continue to site specific interventions within the broader context of all the potential resources available to people living with HIV.

Notes

1 National comparative data was obtained from the National Survey of Prevalent Diagnosed HIV Infections, Communicable Diseases Surveillance Centre, 1996 (personal communication). This survey is based on reports from clinics in England, Wales and Northern Ireland of their clinic attendees in 1995. It therefore offers a good mapping of the demography of those currently living with an HIV diagnosis. It has two disadvantages: it does not include Scotland (where this data is not collected); and it does not include those who did not attend a clinic in 1995. The national comparisons for place of residence use the report on HIV-1 infected persons by country, region and year of report in the CDSC's AIDS/HIV Quarterly Surveillance Tables (as this includes Scotland).

2 In order to analyze the spread of knowledge among respondents, and to consider possible relationships between knowledge and other questions in the survey, respondents were given 10 points for each of the statements about HIV and AIDS medicine they said they knew. Where someone had disagreed with a statement, the statement was excluded from their overall score; that is, if a respondent disagreed with one statement, they were scored out of the remaining 9; if they disagreed with two statements, they were scored out of the remaining 8. Hence all scores are expressed as percentages. The average score was 56%.

References

ANDERSON, W. and WEATHERBURN, P. (1996) *The Treatment Information Needs of People Living with HIV*. London: NAM Publications.

BAKER, D. and COPELAND, R.A. (1996) 'Treatment education programme for people with HIV-disease'. Paper presented at the XIth International Conference on AIDS, Vancouver (We D3794).

BROWN, G. (1996) 'The HIV/AIDS Treatment Information Network: a community based model for PWAs and their care givers'. Paper presented at the XIth International Conference on AIDS, Vancouver (Mo D235).

GUIMENTO, J. *et al.* (1994) 'Characteristics of users of an AIDS/HIV treatment information resource (the American Foundation for AIDS Research AIDS/HIV Treatments Directory)'. Paper presented at the Xth International Conference on AIDS, Yokohama (PO D3860).

KATZ, D. *et al.* (1996) 'The HIV/AIDS treatment information service: a collaborative US public health service initiative'. Paper presented at the XIth International Conference on AIDS, Vancouver (Tu C212).

KORSIA, S. and MAJCHROWICZ, M. (1994) 'Be good to yourself: a self-care manual providing relevant treatment information to HIV-infected inmates'. Paper presented at the Xth International Conference on AIDS, Yokohama (Po B3378).

KUROMIYA, K. and BAUER, R. (1996) 'Rapid AIDS information dissemination to hard-to-reach communities using the World Wide Web technology'. Paper presented at the XIth International Conference on AIDS, Vancouver (We D3897).

MARK, F. (1994) 'HIV/AIDS treatment information dissemination using a toll-free hotline'. Paper presented at the Xth International Conference on AIDS, Yokohama (P D0182).

MCCLURE, C. *et al.* (1996) 'HIV positive peers as treatment information counsellors: training programme and service delivery'. Paper presented at the XIth International Conference on AIDS, Vancouver (Mo D1785).

MCLANAHAN, S. *et al.* (1994) 'Development of a bibliographic index of non-traditional treatment information sources (by the Haemophilia and AIDS/HIV Network for the Dissemination of information)'. Paper presented at the Xth International Conference on AIDS, Yokohama (PO D4051).

NALBANDIAN, T. *et al.* (1996) 'A national toll-free AIDS hotline staffed entirely by people living with HIV'. Paper presented at the XIth International Conference on AIDS, Vancouver (Th D5111).

PLEASANT, K. *et al.* (1996) 'Project TEACH (Treatment Education Activists Combatting HIV)'. Paper presented at the XIth International Conference on AIDS, Vancouver (We D3784).

THOMAS, J. (1994) 'Current cutting-edge HIV treatment information dissemination through the town meeting forum'. Paper presented at the Xth International Conference on AIDS, Yokohama (PD0181).

Notes on Contributors

Will Anderson is currently a research associate at Sigma Research, University of Portsmouth, where he is engaged in quantitative and qualitative research into the social aspects of HIV treatment. His experience of HIV treatment information work was gained as director of NAM Publications, publisher of the *National AIDS Manual* and *AIDS Treatment Update*.

Peter Aggleton is Professor in Education and Director of the Thomas Coram Research Unit at the Institute of Education, University of London. He has worked internationally in HIV/AIDS health promotion since the mid-1980s. His publications include *Health* (Routledge, 1990), *AIDS: Activism and Alliances* (edited, with Peter Davies & Graham Hart, Taylor & Francis, 1997), *Success in HIV Prevention* (AVERT, 1997); and *Men who Sell Sex* (edited, UCL Press, 1998).

Carolyn Baylies is a senior lecturer in sociology at the University of Leeds. She has carried out research in Zambia on electoral politics, class formation and the state and democratization, and has also published work on indigenous enterprise, gender and health.

Susan Beardsell was a senior research fellow with Sigma Research based in London when this research was conducted. She subsequently worked as a commissioning development adviser with the Substance Misuse Advisory Service and is now a freelance researcher based in Brighton.

Eddy Beck is senior lecturer in epidemiology and public health at Imperial College School of Medicine, St Mary's Campus. His main interests are in assessing the acceptability and cost-effectiveness of health care provision. He was instrumental in setting up the National Prospective Monitoring System on the Use, Cost and Outcome of HIV Service Provision in English Hospitals.

Mary Boulton is senior lecturer in sociology as applied to medicine at Imperial College School of Medicine, St Mary's Campus. She has been involved in a wide range of research in relation to HIV infection and AIDS, including work on changing sexual behaviour among gay men, bisexual men and families of children with HIV/AIDS. She is also interested in research methods and edited *Challenge and Innovation: Methodological Advances in Social Research on HIV/AIDS* (Taylor & Francis, 1994).

Janet Bujra is a senior lecturer in the Department of Peace Studies, at the University of Bradford. She has carried out research in Tanzania and Kenya on domestic service, prostitution, labour migration, housing and political action, and has also published work on gender, class, ethnicity and economic development.

Danielle Campbell was a research officer at the National Centre in HIV Social Research at Macquarie University, Australia. She is currently enjoying a working holiday in the UK.

Martha Chinouya-Mudari is an African families researcher carrying out doctoral studies at the University of North London (UNL).

Rosalind Coleman has worked in South Africa for four years, most recently with support groups for HIV positive people, and community-based HIV education.

June Crawford is a research consultant to the National Centre in HIV Social Research at the University of New South Wales, Australia, where she has been involved in HIV/AIDS research since 1987. Her background is in social psychology and research methodology. She currently divides her research interests between the Sydney Men and Sexual Health (SMASH) cohort study and the Male Call national telephone surveys of gay and homosexually active men.

Peter Davies is the co-author of *Sex, Gay Men and AIDS* (Falmer Press, 1993), and editor with Peter Aggleton and Graham Hart of many books in the Social Aspects of AIDS series.

Catherine Donovan is a lecturer in sociology at Sunderland University. She has researched and published in the areas of reproductive technologies, AIDS/HIV, and lesbian and gay relationships.

Kevin Eisenstadt was a research fellow at South Bank University, where he conducted the research described here. He is now working in HIV prevention with gay men for a local authority in London.

Paul Flowers is a sexual health research fellow at the MRC Medical Sociology Unit, University of Glasgow. He is currently involved in the design and evaluation of an intervention involving gay men and their HIV risk-related behaviours.

Judy French is a research officer at the National Centre in HIV Social Research at the University of New South Wales, Australia. She has been involved in sexuality and HIV/AIDS research since 1992.

Philip Gatter is a senior research fellow in the Social Sciences Research Centre at South Bank University, London. He has worked on the evaluation of HIV/AIDS social care services, and is currently writing a book called *Identity and Sexuality: AIDS in Britain in 1990s* (to be published by Cassell).

Graham Hart is assistant director of the MRC Medical Sociology Unit, University of Glasgow, where he directs a programme of research on sexual and reproductive health. He has undertaken studies of risk in gay men, injecting drug users and sex workers, and published widely in the HIV/AIDS field. He is co-editor of the journal *AIDS Care*, and general editor of the *Health, Risk and Society* (UCL Press) series of books.

Brian Heaphy is a research fellow in the Social Science Research Centre at South Bank University, London. He is currently completing research on the changing identities of people living with AIDS/HIV, and is working on various publications concerning non-heterosexual relationships with Catherine Donovan and Jeffrey Weeks.

Paul Holland worked for two years as a research associate at Sigma Research, investigating various aspects of HIV and sexual health. He is now working as a senior therapist for the Centre of Education and Intervention in Early Childhood and embarking on a career in neuropsychology.

Peter Keogh was a senior research fellow with Sigma Research, based in London. In addition to this work on HIV positive gay men and a range of pre-testing and evaluation projects, he has worked on a multi-site research and development project on public sex environments and safer sex. He is now a freelance research consultant.

Susan Kippax is director of the National Centre in HIV Social Research at the University of New South Wales, Australia. She has been involved in many aspects of HIV/AIDS research since 1986, and is the author of numerous publications on the social aspects of AIDS. Her publications have appeared in a number of journals, and (with R.W. Connell, G.W. Dowsett and J. Crawford) she is co-author of *Sustaining Safe Sex: Gay Communities Respond to AIDS*, (Taylor & Francis, 1993).

David Miller is Emeritus Professor of Public Health Medicine at Imperial College School of Medicine and is an honorary senior research fellow in the Department of Public Health at UMDS. His main interests have been in the epidemiology of infectious diseases, particularly acute respiratory infections in children, and immunization.

Margaret O'Brien is Professor of Family Studies and Head of the School of Social Work at the University of North London (UNL).

Katy Pepper is currently working as a social development advisor on the Nepal Safer Motherhood Project. She has a background in nursing and trained in anthropology at Oxford University.

Garrett Prestage is a project scientist at the National Centre in HIV Epidemiology and Clinical Research at the University of New South Wales, Australia. He has been involved in social research within the Sydney gay community since 1982, and in HIV research and prevention since 1984. He coordinates the Sydney Men and Sexual Health cohort study and co-edited *Sex Work and Sex Workers* (University of NSW Press, 1994).

Gill Seidel is a social scientist and discourse analyst interested in the construction of marginality. She has been working on gender and HIV/AIDS in sub-Saharan Africa (Uganda, Nigeria and South Africa) since 1987.

Jonathan Shepherd is research fellow in the Health Education Unit at the University of Southampton. He has conducted research into the effectiveness of peer-led HIV prevention with young gay and bisexual men. His research interests include evidence-based health promotion, and the effective components of HIV prevention interventions involving gay and bisexual men, women and young people.

Glenn Turner is a senior health promotion specialist at Southampton Health Promotion Services. His research in the field of HIV and sexual health has included a survey of HIV education in further education colleges, a survey of the health needs of gay and bisexual men in Southampton and southwest Hampshire and (with Jonathan Shepherd) an investigation into peer-led HIV prevention with young gay and bisexual men. He is currently involved in research into the characteristics of effective health promotion peer educators.

Paul Van de Ven is deputy director of the National Centre in HIV Social Research at the University of New South Wales, Australia. His current research is on gay men, sexuality and HIV/AIDS. Recent publications have appeared in *AIDS, AIDS Education and Prevention, AIDS Care*, the *International Journal of STD and AIDS*, and the *Journal of Sex Research*.

Sam Walters is senior lecturer in paediatric infectious disease at Imperial College School of Medicine, St Mary's Campus. He trained in paediatrics at

Great Ormond Street Hospital and spent five years working as a paediatrician in Papua New Guinea. Since 1990 he has been primarily involved in providing care to children with HIV infection.

Katherine Weare is a senior lecturer and director of the Health Education Unit at the University of Southampton. Her particular interests are in mental and emotional health, on which she has undertaken research and produced teaching strategies and materials. She is author of the forthcoming book *Promoting Mental and Emotional Health in Schools: Empowerment and Effectiveness* (to be published by Routledge).

Peter Weatherburn is the manager of Sigma Research, a social research group which specializes in the behavioural and policy aspects of HIV and AIDS. Based in south London, the work of Sigma Research focuses increasingly on action research and development projects in collaboration with service providers in the fields of HIV prevention, care and support.

Jeffrey Weeks is Professor of Sociology and Head of the School of Education, Politics and Social Science at South Bank University, London. He is the author of numerous articles and various books on the history and social organization of sexuality. Among his publications are *Coming Out: Homosexual Politics in Britain from the Nineteenth Century to the Present* (Quartet 1977, 2nd edn, 1990); *Sex, Politics and Society* (Longman, 1981, 1989); *Sexuality and its Discontents* (Longman, 1985); *Sexuality* (Routledge, 1986); *Against Nature* (Rivers Oram Press, 1991); *Invented Moralities* (Polity, 1995); and *Sexual Cultures* (edited with Janet Holland, Macmillan, 1996).

Index

abantu 59
access, public sex environments and 125
Adelaide, gay communities in 100
Africa 2, 22
  KwaZulu-Natal (KWZ) 53–65
  Tanzania 35–43, 50–1
  Zambia 35–7, 43–51
African National Congress (ANC) 61
Africans (London)
  networks 114
  refugees 1, 21–33
  use of herbal medicines 13
age
  and HIV prevalence (KwaZulu-
    Natal) 53, 55
  and HIV risk 147–61
  and importance of anal
    intercourse 153–4
  and migration 106–7
  and numbers of partners 153–4
  and status of relationship 154–6
agreements about sex 133–46
  see also negotiated safety
AIDS Council of New South Wales
  158
AIDS Treatment Update 201
AIDS/HIV
  and families of choice 73–5
  people with
    child carers of 21–33
    children 5–20
    disclosure *see* disclosure
    treatment education 199–211
  see also HIV status; interventions;
    prevalence; prevention; testing
alcohol, use of 152–3, 157
alienation, feelings of 147

alternative therapies 13
altruism, motivation of peer educators
  and 165
amyl nitrate (poppers) 153
anal intercourse
  agreements about 133–46
  importance of 153–4
  and status of relationship 74, 154–6
  see also unsafe sex
analytic-inductive methodology 123
anti-HIV therapy
  drugs for 3, 12–13, 206–7
  knowledge of 206–7
  reasons for starting 202–4
  see also treatment education
antibacterial drugs 12
antibiotics 12–13
anxiety, parents' 8–9, 14–15, 19
aromatherapy 13
Asians (Britain) 104, 114
asylum seekers 23
  see also refugees
attitudes
  parents' positive approach 13–14
  peer-led change 174
Australia
  and age 2–3, 147–61
  agreements about sex in 133–46
  gay communities in 99–100
Avon Cemetery 123
AZT 12, 13, 207

Barker, C. 35
Barnados Positive Options 30
bars *see* gay bars
behaviour
  and HIV testing 185, 188–95

and normative values 83–4
see also safer sex; unsafe sex
Big Issue 186
bisexual men, peer-led prevention and
    163–83
bitchiness in gay bars 91–2
blame, apportioning (Africa) 39
blood transfusions and products 5
Boal, Arturo 60
Body Positive 186
Body Positive Newsletter 201
Boulton, M. 99
BRASH 149
Brazil, drama in 60
Brazilians (London) 103–4, 106, 114
Brisbane 149, 152, 158
Britain
    London *see* London
    non-heterosexual family formations in
        67–82
    peer-led HIV interventions in 163–83
        and gay bars 83–98
    treatment education in 199–211
Brixton 107, 108, 115

caregiver's burden 27
carers
    children as 21–33
    friends as 67
    need for, exceeds government and
        NGO services 53
    women expected to be 53, 55, 59
Caribbeans (London) 103, 114
caring for ill people
    in the gay community 75–6
    in village Africa 39, 42
casual partners
    agreements about 139, 142, 144
    and condom use 134, 140–1, 156
    incidence of 137, 157
celibacy, test results and 189
childhood
    of child carers 28–9, 31
    models of 21, 22
childhood illnesses 10–11
children 45
    African refugee 1, 21–33
    as carers 21–33
    and domestic economy 21

with HIV infection 5–20
HIV status in families 26
see also Street Kids
Children Act (1989) 30
choice *see* families of choice
cities
    gay life in 102
    see also Adelaide; Brisbane; Glasgow;
        London; Melbourne; San
        Francisco; Sydney
clubs *see* gay bars and clubs
Colombians (London) 114
combination therapy 199, 200
coming out, family reaction to 69–70
commitment in families 72–3
communications, public sex
        environments and 126–30
community 1
    gay *see* gay community
    lack of support (KwaZulu-Natal) 59
    location of 115
community mobilization 50
    see also mobilization
compartmentalizing life 112–13
concordant relationships *see*
        seroconcordance
condom use
    and casual partners 156
    in gay bars 93–4
    in regular relationships 154–5
    see also safer sex
Continuum 201
cottages 121–32
counselling, role of 187, 194
couple relationships 71, 79
cruising areas 121–32
culture, child carers and 22, 28, 30–1
Cypriots (London) 114

Davies, P. 113
deaf gay men 113
death, denial of friends at 77–8
demographics
    and HIV risk 149–51, 157
    and HIV/AIDS distribution 22–3
Development Bank of South Africa 53
disability, gay community and 113–14
disclosure
    of children's illness (UK) 14–17, 18

and gender (KwaZulu-Natal) 53–65
of parents' illness (UK) 25, 28
in storytelling (KwaZulu-Natal) 58–9
discordant relationships
   agreements in 138–41
   definition of 134
   see also HIV status
doctors
   and decisions about anti-HIV therapy
      202–3, 204, 206, 207–9
   and children 12–13
   as information sources 204–5
Dowsett, G. 99
drama
   forum theatre 60, 61
   Muchinka Women's Drama Group
      45, 46–7, 49, 50
drugs
   anti-HIV *see* anti-HIV therapy
   recreational 152–3, 157

education
   and HIV risk 149–50, 157
   migration for 103–5
   in peer-led interventions 173–4
   treatment education 199–211
   see also school
education programmes, regional
      variations in 158
employment, HIV risk and 150
empower women slogan 35
esoteric sex 157, 159
ethnic background
   and gay community 114–15
   and migration in Britain 104
   of parents of sick children 7, 8
   of UK population 23
evaluation in peer-led initiatives 168,
      170–5, 177–8
   training 165–6
extended families 67
   see also non-heterosexual family
      formations

families 1
   and children with HIV 5–20
   of choice *see* families of choice
   definitions of 67
   HIV status in 26

non-heterosexual 67–82
one-parent 17, 19, 23, 30
of origin *see* families of origin
pretended families 68
and refugees child carers 1, 21–33
   disruptions to 29–30
   response to disclosure 15, 17
   see also children
families of choice 67–75
   see also non-heterosexual family
      formations
families of origin 72
   denial of friends by 77–8
   response to partners 78
   see also families
feeding HIV infected children 11–12
Fern Park 124, 128
forum theatre 60, 61
   see also drama
Freirian techniques 60
friends
   as family 71
   networks of 112–13
   and the value of relationships 76–9
   see also non-heterosexual family
      formations
funerals 78–9

gay bars and clubs 108–12
   disability and ethnicity 113–15
   health promotion in 116–17
   and peer-led intervention 83–98
gay community
   age and involvement in 151–2
   caring in 74–6
   disability in 113–14
   ethnicity in 114–15
   peer-led interventions in 83–98
   understanding required of 99–100
Gay and Lesbian Mardi Gras Fair Day
      134
gay men
   agreements about sex 133–46
   in cottages and cruising areas 121–32
   and HIV risk
      and age 147–61
      and HIV testing 185–98
   and non-heterosexual family
      formations 67–82

peer-led work 163–83
  and gay bars 83–98
  social networks of 99–120
  and treatment education 199–211
Gay Men Fighting AIDS (GMFA) 101,
  180
gay venues *see* gay bars and clubs
gender
  and blame 39
  and disclosure through storytelling
    53–65
  and expectations of care 27
  and HIV prevalence 53–4, 55
  improvements in relations 48
  and mobilizing women (Africa) 35–52
  see also men; women
generational differences (Africa) 42, 43
Geneva Convention (1951) 23–4
Giddens, A. 74
girls, caring by (UK) 25–30
Glasgow, peer-led work in 83–98
globalization, challenging 61
GMFA (Gay Men Fighting AIDS) 101
gossip, gay bars and 91–2
guilt, families with HIV and 18, 26

Hackney 23
Hapeer Project 164–6
Hart, G. 99
health status
  and anti-HIV therapy 203–4
  children's 7–11
    family concern over (UK) 18–19
    promoting 11–14
  see also HIV status; treatment
herbal medicines 13
heterosexual men
  gay men's friendships with 112–13
  public sex environments used by 121
  reduced vulnerability of (Africa) 51
heterosexual transmission 22
heterosexuals
  choosing family relationships 71
  disclosure using storytelling (Africa)
    53–65
  men *see* heterosexual men
  and mobilizing women (Africa) 35–52
  and negotiated safety 191
  risk assessment by 192–3

see also sexuality
HIV *see* AIDS/HIV
HIV and Family Life Project 24, 31
HIV positive people as information
  sources 204–5
HIV status 133–4
  and agreements on sex 138–44
  conversion of 6
  distribution in families 26
  and sexual practices 154–6, 158
  and testing behaviour 150–1
  see also health status; testing
homeopathic treatments 13
homosexuals 2
  see also gay men; lesbians; sexuality
Humphrey, L., *Tearoom Trade* 121

identity 115
  see also sexual identity
inductive analysis 7
information sources for HIV
  treatments 204–6
interactive narrative design 58–61
international migration 103–4
  see also refugees
interventions and initiatives
  peer-led 163–83
    and gay bars 83–98
  in Zambia 44–51
  see also prevention
interviews
  with families of children with HIV 6–
    7
  at gay bars 86, 88–9
  and investigating risk taking 186
  in peer-led initiatives 171–7
    and evaluation 178
    follow up 173
    structure of 169–70
intranational migration 104–6
invulnerability, illusions of 147
Ireland, migrants from 106–7
Islington 107
isolation, feelings of 147

Johnson, A. 103

kidembwa 40, 42, 43
knowledge, HIV-related 152, 206–7,

208–9
KwaZulu-Natal (KWZ) 53–65

Lambeth 23, 107
language difficulties, child refugees
    and 25, 29
Latin Americans (London) 114
lesbians
    gay men's friendships with 112–13
    migration to cities 103
    see also non-heterosexual family
        formations
Lewisham 107, 108
life, quality of, for children 14–18
literature, campaigning 35
London
    AIDS conference at 1
    children in
        African refugees 21–33
        with HIV infection in 5–20
    gays in
        cottages and cruising areas 121–
        32
        migration to 102–6
        and social networks 99–120
lone parents 17, 19, 23, 30
love, friendship and 72
Lushoto 37–43, 50–1

McInnes, D. 99
Mainliners 186
Mainliners Newsletter 201
Mansa 43–51
Melbourne
    HIV knowledge in 152
    studies in 148, 149, 157
men
    bisexual 163–83
    gay *see* gay men
    heterosexual *see* heterosexual men
    see also gender; women
migration 100, 102–7, 116
    see also refugees
Mill Street Cottage 123, 128
Miss London 186
MMASH 149
mobility 116
mobilization, women's (Africa) 35–
    52

mobilize communities slogan 35
motivation, peer educators' 165, 166
Muchinka Women's Drama Group 45,
    46–7, 49, 50
multiple losses 29–30

narratives *see* storytelling
National AIDS Manual (NAM) 199
Natweshe Women's Club 45, 47–8,
    49–50
needs and peer-led initiatives 167, 168,
    176
negative tests, response to 189–91,
    192–3
    see also testing
negotiated safety 141–3
    following testing 190–1
    and heterosexuals 191
    perceived as foolproof 194
    see also agreements
negotiations, difficulties with 174–5
networks
    of friends 112–13
    and gay men 147
        disability and ethnicity 113–15
        and HIV prevention 99–120
        socializing 108–12, 116
    and migration 100
    refugee child carers miss 25, 27–30
    women's (*kidembwa*) 40, 42, 43
New South Wales, studies in 147
newsletters as information sources 204–
    5
non-concordant relationships 134, 138–
    41
    see also HIV status
non-heterosexual family formations
    67–82
normal life, importance of, for children
    14–19
normative values and influence 83–4,
    91–2
North America
    studies on age, and risk 147
    see also USA

obligation in families 72–3
occupation, HIV risk and 150, 157
one-parent families 17, 19, 23, 30

outreach
  and peer-led initiatives 168–9
  questions over 121

parents
  children care for 21–33
  gay 68, 79
  see also families
parks, cruising in 126
  see also public sex environments
participant observation at gay bars 85,
    87
partners
  casual *see* casual partners
  numbers of 137, 152, 153–4
  regular *see* regular partners
PCP prophylaxis 206
PCR tests 206
peer educators, recruiting and training
    164–6
peer-led intervention 3
  and gay bars 83–98
  a new method of 163–83
personal growth, motivation of peer
    educators and 165
pharmacists as information sources 205
Plummer, K. 68, 101
policy makers 30–1, 60
poppers (amyl nitrate) 153
positive approach, parents' 13–14, 19
Positive Speakers 57
positive tests, response to 188–9, 191–2
  see also testing
poverty
  and HIV children (UK) 18
  and HIV/AIDS distribution
    (global) 22
pretended families 68
prevalence of HIV 22–3
  in KwaZulu-Natal (South Africa) 53–
    4, 55
  in Lushoto (Tanzania) 37–8
  in Mansa (Zambia) 44
  and sexual identity (Britain) 163
prevention
  and HIV testing 188
  peer-led 163–83
  in public sex environments 121
  and social networks 99–120

  see also interventions and initiatives
privacy, public sex environments and
    125
proximity, public sex environments
    and 125
public health, HIV testing and 185, 194–
    5
public sex environments (PSEs) 2, 121–
    32
public toilets 121–32
published information as information
    source 205

quality of life 14–18
Queensland AIDS Council 158

Railway Sidings 123–4, 128, 129
Reconstruction and Development
    Programme 61
recruiting peer educators 164–6, 178–9
reflexology 13
Refugee Council 24
refugees 21–33
  definitions of 23–4
  see also migration
regular partners 154–5, 157
  and agreements on sex 137–8
rejection of HIV infected children 15
religious leaders, attitudes of (Africa) 39
reputation, gay bars and 91–2, 93
residential areas (London) 107–8
resourcing, AIDS initiatives and 45, 47
rights and sexuality 79
risk
  assessment of (Africa) 37–8
  HIV 23–4, 147–61
    and testing 187–8
    understanding of 99–100
  social, and public sex environments
    128
Rwandans 24

safer sex
  and age 147–8
  agreements about 133–46
  difficulty maintaining 179
  following HIV testing 188–90
  and status of relationships 74
  see also condom use; unsafe sex

San Francisco, gay families in 67
school
 child carers miss 25, 26, 29
 disclosure to 15, 16
 importance of, for HIV children 14
 lack of gay sex education 163
 see also education
Scotland, peer-led work in 83–98
Septrin 12, 13, 206
seroconcordance
 and agreements 138–41, 190–2
 defined 133
 and sexual activity 154–6, 158
 see also HIV status
sex
 agreements about 133–46
 anal *see* anal intercourse
 open discussion of (Africa) 38–9, 42–3
 in public sex environments (Britain)
  129–32
 safe *see* safer sex
 see also behaviour
sex workers, unprotected sex and 193
sexual identity
 and age 151–2
  development of 156–7
 and agreements on sex 137–8
 and HIV prevalence 163
 see also heterosexuals; homosexuals;
  identity; sexuality
sexual risk
 and testing 185–98
 understanding of 99–100
 see also risk
sexual violence, HIV risk and 24
sexuality
 impact of HIV diagnosis 194
 and rights 79
 socialization of 100, 105
 see also sexual identity
Sigma Research 199
silence, culture of 41
single parents 17, 19, 23, 30
SMASH 149
Social Aspects of AIDS, conference on
 1
social class (London) 107
social constructionism 115
social groupings at gay bars 90–5

social networks *see* networks
social predetermination 124–5, 126–30
social risks in public sex
  environments 128
socialization of sexuality 100, 105
socializing
 and child carers 25, 26, 27, 29
 and gay networks 108–12
 and HIV children 14–18
Soho 101, 107, 109
South Africa 53–65
South Bank University 1
Southampton, University of 164
Southampton Gay Men's Health
  Project 164
Southwark 23
spatial predetermination 124, 125, 126–
  30
storytelling
 functions of narratives 56–7
 interactive narrative design 58–61
 pilot programme using 53–65
Street Kids 45, 48, 49, 50
subversion of public spaces 124
surveys
 at gay bars 85–6, 87–8
 of London gays 101–2
 on sexual agreements 134
Sydney
 gay communities in 100
 gay men's agreements about sex in
  133–46
 health studies in 148, 149
 HIV knowledge in 152
Sydney Gay Community Periodic Survey
  134, 145
symbolic interactionism 115

Tanzania 35–43, 50–1
targeting, peer-led initiatives and 167,
  176
TB, disclosure of 59
testing, HIV 185–98
 and age 150–1
 and behaviour change 188–95
 see also HIV status
Theatre of the Oppressed 60
Time Out 186
toilets 121–32

training peer educators 164–6
transformation, interventions and 36–7, 51
treatment education 199–211
trust
  and friendship families 72
  in relationships 74
Turks (London) 114

Ugandans (London) 24
UNDP (United Nations Development Programme) 44, 46
United Nations Convention on the Rights of the Child 22, 31
United Nations Development Programme (UNDP) 44, 46
United Nations High Commission for Refugees 24
unsafe sex
  agreements about 133–4, 138–44
  discussions of, in peer-led interventions 174–5
  and female sex workers 193
  incidence of 163
  reasons for 190–3, 194
  and status of relationship 74, 154–7
  see also safer sex
USA
  gay families in 74
  migration by gay men in 102

and peer-led intervention 84
  see also North America

vertical transmission 5, 22
violence, sexual, and HIV risk 24
voluntary work, resourcing, and AIDS initiatives 45

war and civil strife 24, 29–30
withdrawal, beliefs about 152, 158
women
  as carers 27, 53, 55, 59
    girls (UK) 25–30
  disclosure
    rejection following (Africa) 55–6
    through storytelling (Africa) 53–65
  diversity of interests 35–6
  gay men's friendships with 112–13
  networks (*kidembwa*) 40, 42, 43
  risk assessment by 192–3
  sex workers 193
  status and rights (Africa) 39
  see also gender; men
workshops (Africa) 41–3

youth, HIV risk and 147–61

Zairians (London) 24, 25–6
Zambia 35–7, 43–51